TO HEAL
A NATION

The One-Hundred-Year Lifestyle

Life choices with proven effectiveness for better
physical, mental, and spiritual health.
Learn how to live the wellness lifestyle in the drug-free zone.

Spinal neglect is a pandemic of epic proportions!
Its ignorance that the majority seek out
pharmaceuticals first and chiropractic last.
We need a better collaboration, a global education process is
needed regarding spinal care from the onset of our youth.

**"…and for by Pharmakeia (pharmaceutical),
all nations were deceived." Revelations 18:23**

JEFFREY TRIGO, D.C.

ISBN 978-1-0980-3065-0 (paperback)
ISBN 978-1-0980-4367-4 (hardcover)
ISBN 978-1-0980-3066-7 (digital)

Christian Faith Publishing, Inc.
832 Park Avenue
Meadville, PA 16335
www.christianfaithpublishing.com

Printed in the United States of America

DEDICATION

This book is dedicated to my dad Robert F.S. Trigo, D.C. who adjusted me since my birth and inspired me to follow his footsteps and become a wellness provider and public servant. He was a man of many hats who served in the army in his youth, received a doctor of chiropractic degree in 1967 and was also a pastor, doctor of divinity. He truly had a servant's heart, was a great chiropractor, and American Patriot. He was a true pioneer in Japan by introducing chiropractic education at a very high level in that country, and since that first meeting in 1992, in which I was a part of, there is now over ten thousand chiropractic clinics in Japan and that country is a healthy place to live for it.

Dr. Yasunori Iwama, you are a true visionary and leader. Thank you for the love you showed my father and I. It was a total blessing to travel throughout your great and beautiful country teaching chiropractic to a bunch of excited passionate professionals. I was filled with amazement and awe as I witnessed so much love and passion that your doctors expressed for the chiropractic profession. I have not seen this level of love and excitement demonstrated anywhere else in the world.

And finally to the 600 chiropractors who were jailed for "practicing medicine without a license." Starting with Dr. Reba Willis in 1922 who served 6 months, and ending with Dr. E.J. Mussen who served time in 1975; all jailed for giving a chiropractic spinal adjustment. These legends paved the road for our great profession and preserving our future. Without these pioneers, who kept their pisiforms polished as they stayed connected to the streets, despite the law, the great chiropractic profession would not be where it is today, worldwide!

"You never know how the effects of something you say hear or do will affect the lives of millions tomorrow."
(B. J. Palmer)

Thank you, Dad, for all your love and passion you have shown to our great profession, the torch was passed and it's in good hands! You touched many lives and inspired many to become chiropractors; you were definitely a life changer for many people including myself. Your passion and inspiration toward our great profession was legendary and addictive. I love you; see you in Heaven one day.

In Jesus's name, amen!

Get the big idea and all else follows.
(B. J. Palmer)

I have had the privilege to eyewitness the many lives that our great profession has changed by the gentle, accurate chiropractic adjustment. This adjustment removes nerve interference and restores joint motion by restoring normal position of the spinal column. Longevity and function are the byproduct of a well-adjusted spine; changing fate as we remove the cloak of harm by shifting focus on causation, its removal and cure. It is my wish that no spine gets left behind.

"Fools multiply when wise men are silent." (Nelson Mandela)

"Men of principle are principal men." (B.J. Palmer)

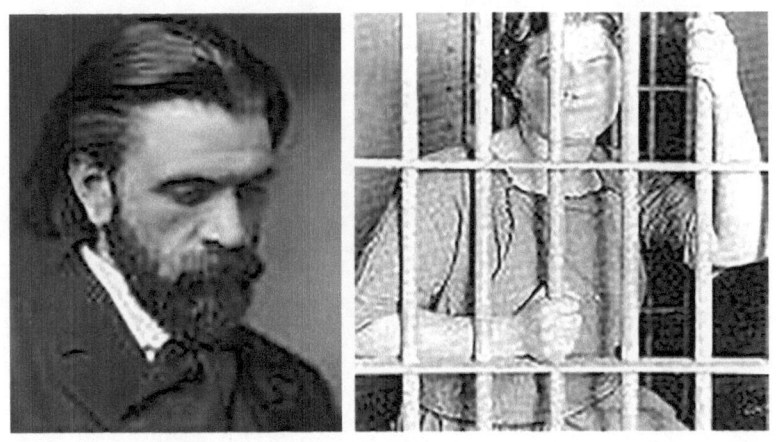

B.J.Palmer, D.C   Put in jail for Chiropractic

**"When Tyranny becomes law rebellion
becomes duty." (Thomas Jefferson)**

CONTENTS

Dedication 3

Introduction..9

Chiropractic History of Jeff Trigo, DC 13

Chapter 1:   Our Inner Healer 17
Chapter 2:   Our Vital Connection 29
Chapter 3:   The Silent Killer.....................................36
Chapter 4:   Toxicities and Deficiencies.........................47
Chapter 5:   Natural Remedies 71
Chapter 6:   Powerful Pisiform 129
Chapter 7:   Against All Odds 149
Chapter 8:   Move Well 165
Chapter 9:   Eat Well 182
Chapter 10: Think Well...200
Chapter 11: Athletic Edge..225
Chapter 12: Children Are People Too 236
Chapter 13: "Big Pharma" 250
Chapter 14: Insurance Ideology 262
Chapter 15: Freedom of Choice.................................270
Chapter 16: Q&A with the Patients.............................287
Chapter 17: Final Exhortations 299

About the Author 307

INTRODUCTION

I was born into a chiropractic family, as a second generation chiropractor and pioneer with my dad in the advancement of this great profession overseas in Japan, I have had the privilege of witnessing so many miracles that it would be sin not to share this with the rest of the world. I am deeply saddened by what is going on in healthcare around the world today. Occasionally, I get a glimmer of hope as we discover scientific health breakthroughs or witness another miracle by the millions within our profession, but overall, I see a broken down and bankrupt failed health care system with flawed ideology and with risky shady results often ending in poor health, worsened conditions, or loss of life.

People are often being prescribed something that would make a well man sick therefore how would one expect to get a sick man well? The amounts of people we lose to death via "modern-day medicine" have reached pandemic proportions and it can't be ignored any longer.

If we can shift our thought (Thot) patterns and start to view our body as an intelligent design, then we can look within ourselves when loss of wellness is present and ask a better question like, "What is our body toxic with, or what is our body deficient with?" If something in the body is toxic, "remove it." If a deficiency is present, then "add it." This scientific sound approach to health care has always yielded faster and safer results, time and time again. True health is expressed physically, mentally, and spiritually; and they all are working simultaneously in harmony together like the Buddy Rich Big Band Orchestra. I will do my best to keep the doctor interested in this read as well as the layperson and use technical scientific or medical terms while always trying to use easy to understand metaphors and analogies thereafter so that any level of the educated persons may have a greater understanding of the underlying message.

It is my hope and desire that the wisdom found in this book would truly educate and bless the lives of millions of people, while preventing unnecessary surgeries, procedures, pills, potions, and lotions from being administered or prescribed. I hope this knowledge goes viral while creating a drastic change in the way people eat, think and move.

I also want to pass along this great wealth of knowledge accumulated over one hundred years by various chiropractic pioneers before my time and my vast experience; to educate the public and change the way they view loss of wellness and the expression of dis/ease, a B.J. Palmer term, and the incredible and remarkable ways their body can heal itself. I hope to remove old ways of thinking and create new action plans for the suffering while shifting millions toward wellness absent of dis-ease and ailment. I hope that millions of people would experience a greater quality of life for all who implement this wellness lifestyle. Imagine living life decade after decade with literally zero dis/ease or symptoms, truly thriving physically, mentally, and spiritually. This will compound life's joy exponentially.

Health is a choice, and it doesn't happen by chance. Take charge of your life today; become the author of your own health and wellness destiny.

Learn how not to become a victim with a disease story, but rather experience all that life has to offer you. Health and wellness is compounded over time and within the chapters of this book you will learn lifestyle changes that can take you beyond the triple digits.

Please be open to a change in the way you think, because God doesn't make junk. We all have a doctor within us that is truly trying to express life at its maximum.

Each chapter will act as a building block showing evidence towards intelligent design, with easy, safe and effective treatment methods that yield powerful results that you will really enjoy. This concept towards change can heal a nation, making America healthy again.

Prevention is the key and the earlier you implement the changes the more health benefits you will reap. Knowledge is power! Many areas of your life like your health, finances, relationships, physical-mental-spiritual health, fitness levels, etc., can all experience the rewards of the compound effect in these areas of your life. You will learn many different valuable tools throughout the contents of this book to lead you towards a healthier, well-balanced life.

I look forward to seeing the change in the world, one spine at a time.

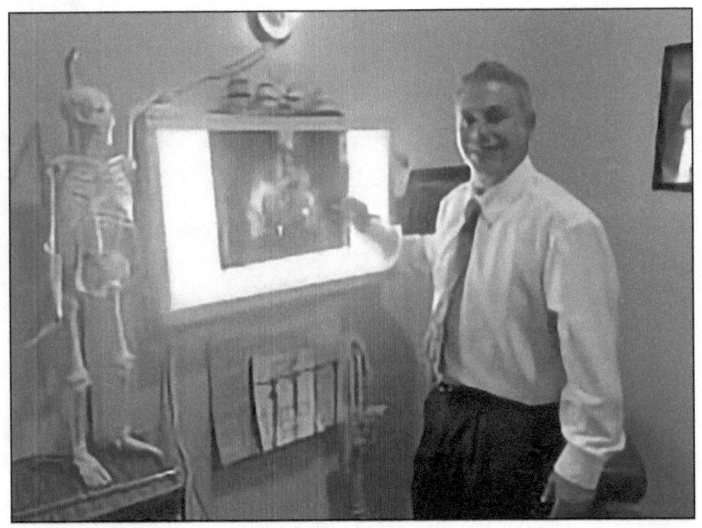

God bless you always.
Jeffrey Trigo, D.C., C.M.E.
www.TrigoChiropractic.com

Chiropractic History of Jeff Trigo, DC

When I was born, my dad was already in chiropractic school learning how to adjust the spine. A chiropractic adjustment helped him with his back pain, so he wanted to do that for others. Therefore, I'm a second-generation chiropractor with the hope that one of my children will also become a chiropractor making us a rare third generation of chiropractors in the family. I was fortuitous by being a chiropractic baby, and I have been adjusted for my whole life. I remember getting pulled out of line in the eighth grade when they were handing out vaccinations filled with undisclosed ingredients that they wanted to inject directly into your kid's blood stream thus bypassing all normal portals of entry. Those that were giving the shots pulled me out of line and said, "Your dad is a doctor, and he has you taken care of. This shot is not for you," as I watched all my friends getting in line and getting a shot in the arm, I began to contemplate and wonder why not me!

I went home and asked my dad that day what was this all about, and that's when he started explaining the philosophy of chiropractic—about our "inner healer" and "innate wisdom," etc. I remember when my dad came home after a long day of work, he was hurting sometimes and would ask me to adjust him after demonstrating what he wanted me to do on my sister. I would then try it on him, and he would say things like, "Drop your elbow a bit," or "More speed," "Push like this," "Hold your hand like that," etc. I learned how to start adjusting some areas of the spine at the age of fifteen, that's a young age to start "practice." I would adjust neighbors, friends, family members—never got paid of course. After years of various jobs and diagnostic technician certifications, I went to school to become a chiropractor. In school, I was class representative. I was named the guy who would go the extra mile "extra miler" for his peers award. I also was the only trimester 2 student allowed to mentor trimester 1 classmates every trimester till I graduated.

Gifted with an overseas chiropractic teaching relationship that my father built prior to my graduation, I went to school with a different mind-set than that most of my peers. I went with a notion that I, too, would be teaching chiropractic overseas in Japan—therefore learn as much technique as you can while in school. I would stay later to go to the adjusting clubs. Pick my clinician's mind about technique, etc. At a young age, I learned the importance of regular care. I stopped getting sick (flus and colds) and decades would go by without illness. If I got a sinus infection, I got adjusted and it went away. I got hurt in a slide tackle in AYSO when I was twelve, a hip and lumbar adjustment got me back the very next game playing at 100 percent. I suffered from bad headaches from a bike injury that knocked me out, and I woke up in the hospital. Disabling migraines started to plague me, then my dad, when he got back to town, divorced and living in Hawaii, adjusted me, and poof, my migraines were gone. He then made sure I had a local chiropractor available to me at all times that I could see because he always lived so far away and regular care was impossible otherwise. Any time I suffered from heartburn, the adjustment restored normal function and the symptom again disappeared.

Time after time, these adjustments were restoring life in my body and the normal return of function was being restored naturally; therefore, this made me start to contemplate becoming a chiropractor like my dad so that I can be used by God to do His healing also.

I started pre-chiropractic courses at the age of twenty-eight and received my doctor of chiropractic degree at age thirty-four in 1999. Ever since then, I've been connected to the streets telling everyone about the healing powers of the chiropractic adjustment.

God doesn't make junk, and He really wants the best for you; therefore, He uses people like me to correct and remove the source of so many unwanted conditions that are plaguing people worldwide.

Wellness is a choice; it doesn't happen by chance. I will teach you how to eat well, motivate you to get the body of yours exercising, and if you take care of your spine, it will take great care of you!

Jeff Trigo, DC
www.TrigoChiropractic.com
Dr.JeffTrigo@hotmail.com

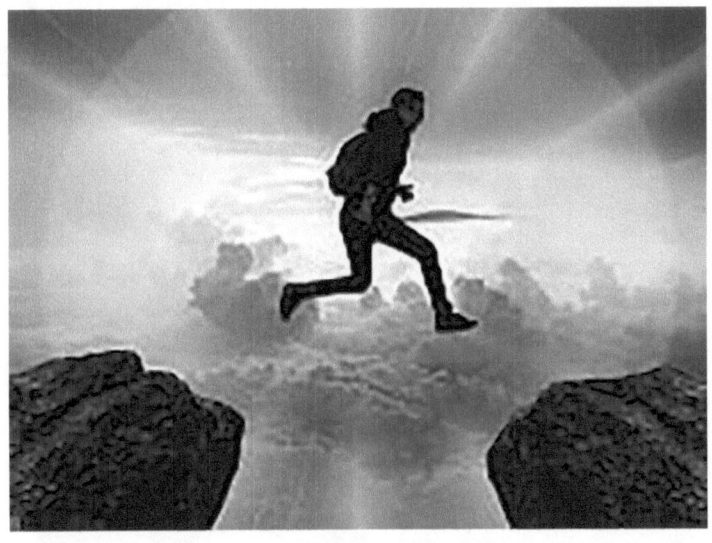

Time to shift our thought patterns towards Devine Design

"For I will restore health to you and heal you of your wounds, says the Lord…" Jeremiah 30:17

**Beloved, I pray that you may prosper in all things and be in health, just as your soul prospers.
3 John 1:2**

CHAPTER 1

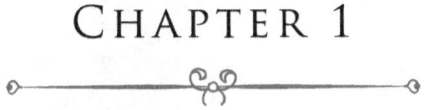

Our Inner Healer

Our inner healer is absolutely remarkable! It is the life force within us that provides all living creatures with that internal wisdom to govern or function, to survive, adapt, metabolize. A built-in power source designed to last up to 120 years, what a design. Feed it correctly and extend your years while slowing down the aging process. Move it well and see energy like you've never seen before. Keep all function at "power on" status and experience wellness not only absent of dis/ease but truly thrive! What a machine our body is remarkable in design wonderfully made in its design indeed.

This governing entity within us is often referred to as innate wisdom, and it is bestowed upon us as a gift from universal intelligence. This gift from God, embedded in our DNA, allows innate to have its very own regulatory agency and/or auto pilot completely controlled and under coordination via our brain, spinal cord, and all of its nerves, AKA the master system.

The master system operates a lot like the electrical company does, sending out cords and wires to provide power and energy to every electrical gadget in our community, towns, and homes. Well, the same is true for the nervous system.

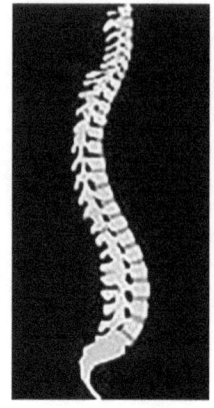
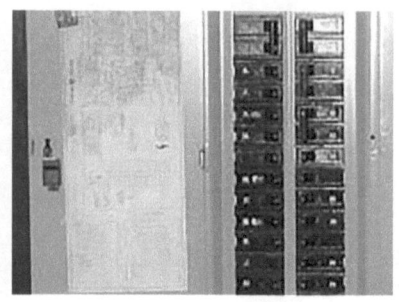
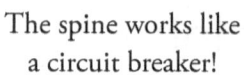
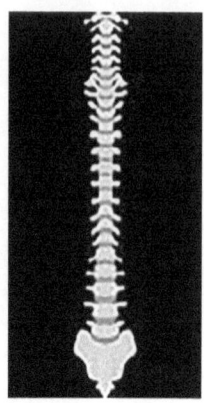

The spine works like
a circuit breaker!

**"The brain, spinal cord and nerves control and
coordinate all organs and structures of the human body."
(Gray's Anatomy, Twenty-Ninth Edition, page 4)**

I have this book in my collection and it used to belong to Carl Cleveland Jr., DC. It's signed by him, a second-generation chiropractor like myself. He continued with his dad's legacy of training doctors of chiropractic throughout various campuses. I attended the Los Angeles campus from April 1996 to August 1999. When they closed the LA location, they sold books in their library, and I found this little jewel! The reason I mention all this is because you can no longer find this abovementioned quote in the Gray's Anatomy later editions or in other anatomy books today. Why? Has the body changed or is there a "special interest" in preventing this information to reach those who study anatomy today?

It would seem that hiding this information from the new and upcoming doctors attending schools today could prevent a huge awareness which may prove to cause a drop in drug sales and expose the truth about how our bodies really work. In other words, don't let the public know how the body is under direct control of the nervous system, and we can really profit from their sickness care! You will read more on this later.

"Look well to the spine for the cause of disease." (Hippocrates, The Father of Chiropractic, not The Father of Medicine) FYI dear readers, he has many nutritional and spinal wellness quotes that support this, not talks of medicine etc.

The Pathway of the Master System is above, down, from the inside-out (ADIO). Above is the brain, traveling down is the spinal cord, and exiting the spine from the inside-out are the nerves. These nerves travel through the intervertebral foramina (IVF) exiting the spine and travel to thousands of destinations. That is how the body heals. Inside-out! Nerves are made up of neurons a specialized conductor cell that receives and transmits electrochemical nerve impulses. This pathway is a two-way communication highway—brain to tissue cell and tissue cell to brain. Many would have you to believe that the opposite is true; outside-in is how we heal, so that you need something added to your imperfectly and flawed self. If flawed and missing concept is accurate then you must add something to your body to heal it, like a potion, lotion, pills, shots, procedures, bolts, screws, laser beams, and crystal balls. So outside-in concept and theory, that the body is flawed and unintelligent in design therefore we must put something on or in the body has many people fooled. Often we hear about all surgical procedures in which body parts are removed; when in doubt, cut it out! This, of course, yields poor results with many dangerous side effects, while ignoring and failing to locate the cause of the original symptom and fixing it! That's comparable to putting a sticker over your check engine blinking red light on your dash board while driving because that warning light is bothersome and annoying. Who does that? Tens of millions of people daily with their sickness symptoms as Americans and other people of the world "pop pills" by the truck loads!

America counts for only 5 percent of the world's population yet we consume 80 percent of the world's opioids! I wonder why the gullible keep allowing a script pad to be handed to them as they continue popping pills and dying. Is it because they don't know better? It is once again my hope that this book will change that. Allow the shift in the many to change the way they understand physiology and biological function, a.k.a. the study of life. Embrace the knowledge of what causes a man to thrive versus what causes a man to die.

The pill popping becomes very addicting and controlling. The "side effects" are good business, profits up, shareholders happy as sickness care causes big profits to rise; it's evil! Doctors, DO NO HARM! We pledged an oath to do what is in the best interest for the care of the patient.

In fact, a billion dollars are spent each day trying to brainwash you on outside in thinking mentality. This money is spent via TV, cable, radio, billboards, magazines, etc. The investors of this are hopeful that you will run to the pharmacy, buy that gadget or device and spend your hard earned income trying to finally fix the problem you've been suffering with. Poor and shady results are often the byproduct while leaving you needing the next big thing or procedure. All of these poor choices, not finding the cause, often lead to disability, disease, or condition advancement with loss of any quality of life and/or early death.

**"Intelligence is present everywhere in our bodies…
our own inner intelligence is far more superior to
any we can try to substitute from outside…"
(Deepak Chopra, MD)**

**"But now, O LORD, you are our Father; we are the clay, and you
are our potter; we are all the work of your hand." Isaiah 64:8**

**Get wisdom! Get understanding! Do not forget, nor turn
away from the words of my mouth. Do not forsake her,
and she will preserve you; Love her, and she will keep you.
Wisdom is the principal thing; Therefore get wisdom. And
in all your getting, get understanding. Proverbs 4:5–7**

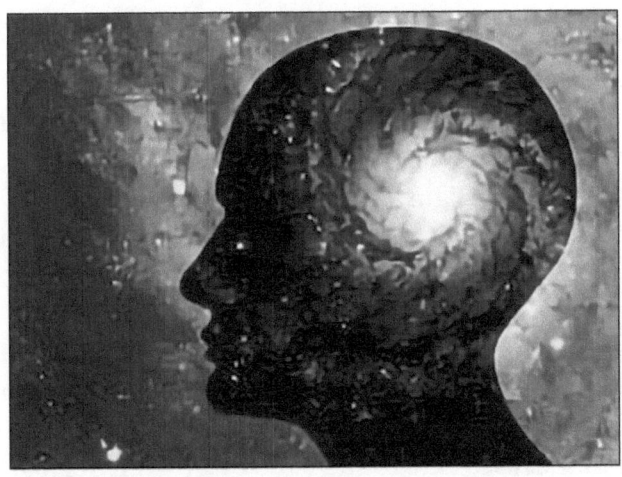

Our inner healer, controlled by these neuro impulses is within us all. We are born with it. It controls every function, and all systems, organs, tissues, cells, glands, muscles, and areas of skin throughout our whole body. We have this inner healer embedded in our DNA, it controls our DNA. Our wonderfully divinely designed and created body with its own innate life force preinstalled before our birth. Our inner healer, the pathway of life is ADIO. It happens no other way! Universal intelligence gifted us with this inner healer we call innate wisdom; it is controlled and governed by our master system with billions of nerve impulses being transmitted simultaneously while regulating bone growth, food processing, hormone production, immune system optimization, reproductive system monitoring, metabolic regulations, etc. Interference to this information highway introduces a lower state of function that is not optimum. A dis/eased state of lowered function often leading to eventual symptoms. Compounded over time this dis/eased state of operation starts to show its ugly head as symptoms start appearing and then the body loses its potential for maximum state of wellness and health. A wonderful example of innate wisdom is the star fish; if one of the star fish's arms breaks off, a new one will grow exactly the same length as the others. Injuries or cuts heal on their own, all growth and regulatory factors are controlled by innate wisdom etc.

With interference to innate, you are no longer performing at peak performance.

Now you are no longer performing at peak performance or at maximum adaptation and weakness or distress sets in as the body expresses its warning signs as symptoms. Now you have your life-force dimmed, lowering function and vitality. This great loss of innate communication creates dis/ease.

"I desire to know why one person was ailing and his associate, eating at the same table, working in the same shop…was not. Why? What difference was there in the two persons that caused one to have [disease] while his partner… escaped? Why?" (D. D. Palmer, considered the founder of Chiropractic) however there is evidence that adjustments to the spine has been going on for over 5000 years.

You can live forty days without food, four days without water, four minutes without air, but you can't even live four seconds without nerve supply. Once you are brain dead, you are a goner. With all the information that has been presented so far, master healer, universal intelligence, innate wisdom, etc., it makes a lot of sense to make sure that these vital connections don't get crushed, compressed, smashed, or "switched off" like a circuit board on the electrical panel. The weight of a nickel, five grams, is enough pressure to cause a lower state of function, thus decreasing the nerve firing potential immensely. In other words, a compressed nerve is like having a car parked on a water hose affecting the water flow. This compression on a nerve often caused by various conditions, addressed in later chapters, leads to a pathological condition of dis/ease dis/order dis/communication dis/function and so forth.

Health is not defined by how you are feeling. You can feel great one day and twenty-four hours later suffer from a cold, flu or even a heart attack. I often say to a patient:

**"It's not how you're feeling that matters most,
but how you're healing." (Jeff Trigo, DC)**

Chiropractic labeled this function, our inner healer as "innate wisdom" the intelligence which governs and organizes all levels of our complex living, adapting, growing and changing to suit the environment while optimizing function and survival.

"The greatest wealth is Health." (Virgil)

Establishing that reconnection between our inner healer and bodies function should be the goal of every chiropractor. How marvelous is that corrective adjustment that turns up the nerve action potential, restoring a complete undistorted message through its pathway thus allowing Innate to freely flow.

That communication highway is so important to start the healing process and stop the dis/ease expression. Life being restored naturally and safe, allowing innate wisdom to function without distortion is what us chiropractors specialize in. In other words we specialize in the removal of vertebral subluxation complex, VSC.

**"People need to stop looking for the magic pill, potion, lotion
or shot. There is no quick fix, wellness has gone renegade
in today's world! Boost your immunity naturally and take
control of your wellness destination today!" Jeff Trigo, D.C.**

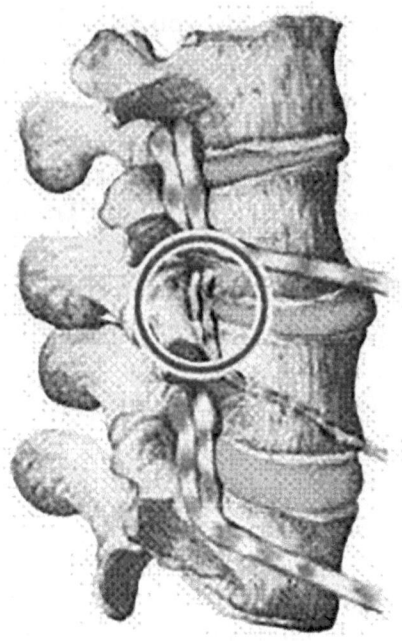

**"Every human being is the author of his
own health or disease." (Sivanada)**

In upcoming chapters you will learn how a very common condition present in all vertebrates, VSC, absolutely shuts down the
ability for innate wisdom to work at optimal levels thus shutting off
our inner healer and diminishing our life force within us. This often
unchecked condition tricks or overwhelms innate wisdom therefore
we lose the ability to thrive. This introduces a lower level of function
within us often called symptoms and/or dis/ease. This inner healer
gets distortion or nociceptor noise that bombards the brain and
fatigues the vertebrate. Failure to thrive is introduced and you may
or may not even feel pain yet. Over time you start waking up sore
and tired. Loss of range of motion creeps in. Popping and clicking
sounds are probably happening now with neck turning or with back
movement. Posture starts distorting and your head goes further and
further forward tightening up your shoulders tighter than a drum!
Sinus or head pressure creeps in, maybe TMJ, shoulder issues, etc.

Maybe digestion and immune system is compromised too as this condition of VSC works its way into multiple levels of your spine granting you an unwanted gift of more and more symptoms. Have you noticed that I never even mentioned low back pain yet? Why? Most people think that the time to visit the chiropractor is when you have back pain, but this is not so. If you have a spine, we all do, it needs maintenance.

The public has been brained washed into thinking that the only reason you should visit a chiropractor is if you have "low back pain"! This should not be so. You have approximately 70 trillion cells in your body, 206 bones, 735 muscles, organs, tissues, glands, etc., all under the direct control of the nervous system and VCS, SHUTS DOWN NERVE FUNCTION! It's really quite simple.

The accurate, gentle precision adjustment to remove subluxation and restore function is an absolute necessity. This action, adjusting vertebra subluxations, needs to be checked from the womb to the tomb. How long do you want 100 percent function in your nervous system, a.k.a. the master system? It makes a great deal of sense to stay regular with your spinal checkups.

Research shows that a subluxation that is two weeks old has already lost its fluid density within the disc visible via MRI. In other words, the white appearance of a hydrated disc is now darker and greyer. Yes, the dehydration process of the disc has already started.

We would never go weeks or months without brushing our teeth, and we can get a new tooth. Why would we go years without an adjustment? There must be a few reasons that I can think of. Fear of the adjustment thinking that it may hurt or become addictive. Ignorance in the fact that you don't know you have subluxation therefore you're chasing symptoms and doing everything under the sun to try and fix oneself instead of finding the cause and removing it. Maybe you heard negative stories spread by the competition that we doctors of chiropractic are quacks. More on that later for sure, it's a great story! Maybe someone you know had a bad experience. Now that person has a polarized opinion that the whole profession is bad therefore even the greatest chiropractic healers don't get a chance to lay hands on their fixations.

I have news for you, if the public in general had a bad experience with a dentist who was subpar, they would absolutely have the wisdom to change dentist and continue caring for their teeth. Chiropractors are not extended that same courtesy. One bad chiropractic experience can cause one patient to be fearful for life and never give it a second chance elsewhere, therefore robbing that person the chance of much needed healing. So now they are jammed or subluxated for life and are only open to hearing treatment options that include pain management, thus ignoring the cause and treating the symptoms with drugs, pills, potions, lotions, bolts, screws, scalpels, electrodes, pins, needles, blue goo, crystal balls, creams, and laser beams.

**"Chiropractic is health insurance.
Premiums small. Dividends LARGE."
(B. J. Palmer)**

Great health is addictive. When you find a great chiropractor, results are swift. It's also good to know that depending on what level of spinal wellness that you present to the doctor of chiropractic, will determine the length of treatment and recovery time needed.

The sooner you start brushing your teeth the healthier your mouth will be. The same is true for your spine. The sooner you start your chiropractic adjustment regimen the less chance of any disc decay or other degenerative arthritic conditions. Remember this,

**"You can get a new tooth but not a new spine.
I wonder why one would neglect something of
such great importance?" (Jeff Trigo, D.C.)**

**"God is the great physician, sometimes He uses people
like chiropractors to bless and heal His people. Tap
into that healing power today." Jeff Trigo, D.C.**

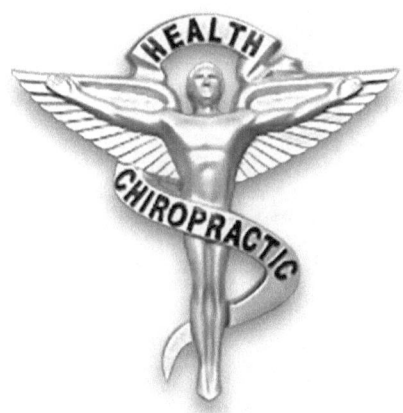

We are programmed from birth to live a healthy long life. It's an accumulation of great life choices in regards to what we eat, think and do that really matter. The treatment of traumatic injuries to our frame must not be ignored, which is the greater controller of lifespan and to the quality of life lived. As you read through the pages of this book, you will continue to learn solid health tips that will absolutely propel you toward the one-hundred-year lifestyle and the sooner you start practicing these wellness principals to your lifestyle, the greater the compound effect of wellness expression in your life you will reap.

And the Lord said, "My Spirit shall not strive with man forever, for he is indeed flesh; yet his days shall be one hundred and twenty years." (Genesis 6:3)

Why are we seeing such short life spans when the Word of God grants us a 120-year life span on this earth? God doesn't make junk! We were created in His own image! We are not supposed to get arthritis and degenerative conditions in our third or fourth decade of life. This is a common but abnormal phenomenon, people! I believe the secrets of longevity are within the pages of this book and I encourage you all to reap the benefits that are revealed within this book. It's a good practice to have zero lag time, so create an action plan that has immediate implementation no matter what age you are currently at. The single most powerful change to your health is the maintenance of 100 percent communication of your inner healer, which governs all function of innate wisdom. When distortion and interference to the intelligence lifeline are restored, expect miracles.

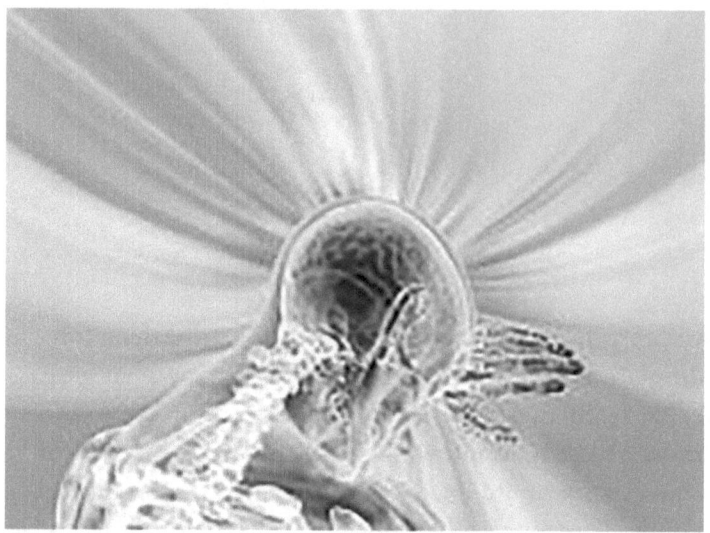

Don't copy the behavior and customs of this world, but let God transform you into a new person by changing the way you think. Then you will learn to know God's will for you, which is good and pleasing and perfect. Romans 12: 2 (NLT)

"People are always more encouraged when we share how God's grace helped us in weakness than when we brag about our strengths." (Rick Warren)

"The earlier abnormal spinal function could be recognized and corrected in a child's life, the greater the opportunity that child will have for neurological development." (Dr. David Heilig)

CHAPTER 2

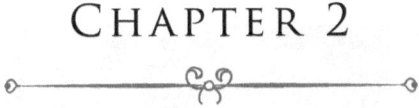

Our Vital Connection

Our vertebral column consists of twenty-four vertebrae plus your sacrum and coccyx. There are thirty-one pairs of spinal nerves that exit the (IVF) and twenty-three discs that act as shock absorbers. Of these twenty-four vertebrae, seven are located in the cervical region (C), with the top bone referred to as C1 the atlas, C2 the axis, then C3–C7 are numbered as such. Twelve vertebrae are located in the thoracic region and have rib attachment sites (T1–T12) with T11 and T12 having floating ribs, not attaching to vertebral bodies. There are five lumbar vertebrae L1–L5, these are the largest and support most of the body's weight. The sacrum is made up of five fused vertebrae, triangular in shape, and it's located at the bottom of the spinal column. The sacrum has articulations with the iliac joint making up the pelvic girdle. The coccyx is at the most inferior (lowest point) area of the sacrum often referred to as the "tailbone." This spinal column primarily serves to house and protect our vital spinal cord and nerves; it has many attachment sites for muscles and ligaments, and adds support for head, shoulders, ribs, and hips. If you look at the spine from front to back, it should be perfectly vertical. Looking at the spine from the side view, lateral, you will see free flowing natural curves existing in a healthy spine. A healthy cervical curve, is approximately 45 degrees, cervical lordosis. A healthy lumbar curve is approximately 36 degrees, lumbar lordosis. The above two mentioned curves are C-shaped. Opposite this C curve would be the angle we see in the

29

thoracic region, it's called kyphosis, and a normal angle is approximately 37 degrees. These normal curves found in the spine along with freely movable joints and lubricated discs act as natural shock absorbers protecting the vital nerves which flow within.

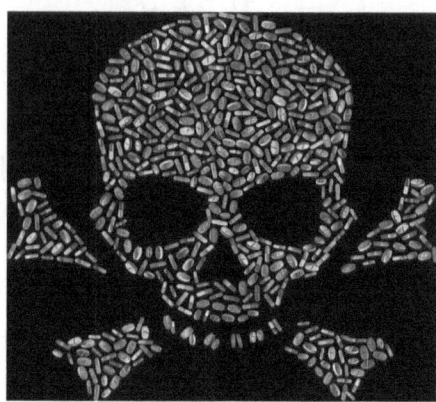

Chasing symptoms or trying to mask them with harmful prescriptions is very risky. It's best to always search for the root cause of the problem. When causation is removed, full function can return. This is imperative for optimal peak performance, absent of dis/ease.

I often demonstrate how our vital connection, communication pathway, can be compromised thus shutting down our innate wisdom between organized function to distorted dysfunction. This demonstration can be observed by twisting and shifting a spinal column. This pathological position reveals a great reduction in size by the IVF, the space where the nerve exits the spine. This closure of the IVF compromises the nerves ability to function at its highest potential. The constant weight or pressure on this nerve forces the wire/nerve, to undergo pathological changes. It loses its proficiency with conduction speed and impulse intensity. An example of this would be demonstrated by having the rubber that wraps a wire wear away and become patchy and scarce. The rubber like material is important for better conduction. The nerve has this wrapping also, it is actually a protein that wraps around the nerve and grows in a spiral pattern completely surrounding the nerve called the myelin sheath. This pathological change, VSC, shrinks (atrophy) the diameter of the nerve and we all know that a smaller wire can't function at the level of a larger gauged wire. You will learn a lot more about the loss of neuroelectrical impulse intensity and the adverse effects it has on our wellness in later chapters as I regularly identify the cause of the dis/ease and offer remedies with proven effectiveness.

To help the patient's memory obtain long term retention on newly taught concepts, I like to use props and visual aids whenever possible. As I twist the spine demonstrating a crushing of the nerve, I simultaneously dim the lights. The dimming of the light correlates with loss of innate wisdom, as vital connection is compromised. In other words, you have a car on a hose and the water just can't freely flow. Only the adjustment will push the bone off the nerve removing causation while restoring function, this is when I turn the lights back to full brightness correlating with the return of their bodies' natural inner healer. I like to congratulate them while informing them that they too have what it takes to truly thrive and live a long healthy drug free life full of vigor.

"Sooner or later the truth comes to light." (Dutch Proverb)

Our spinal column acts like a circuit breaker. If the switch is off and there's no power to the kitchen, do you suggest we run extension cords into the kitchen? Heck no. We will go to our electrical panel and look for the tripped or blown switch and flip it back to the on position, thus "turning the power back on"! A phrase I enjoy using after an adjustment is given to a subluxated spine.

Our nervous system is more remarkable that the vast roadways that stretch out across the great American highways, which many consider a modern marvel. Every cell (approximately 70 trillion) in the body is under direct control of our nervous system. This master system is comprised of trillions of connections and synapses. Nerves are bundled like wires traveling everywhere in and throughout the human design. This vast roadway of nerves acts as a two-way communication highway, able to convey transmissions of energy that control every function from the brain to the tissue cell, and vice versa. The nerves closer to the spine are larger and as they make their way out to organs, tissues, muscles, glands and cells, they get smaller and smaller ending up on the surface of your skin somewhere a.k.a. dermatomes.

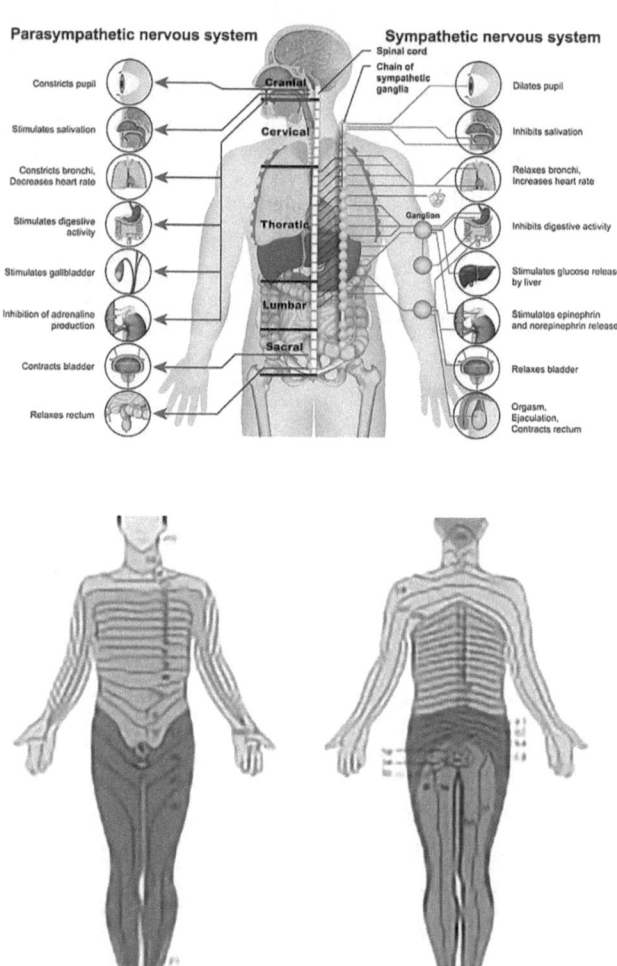

While our vital connection is in full function, thousands of neuro-electrical impulses are being transmitted to every part of our body. Some signals inhibit while others excite. Tens of thousands of programs are in simultaneous operation like one great master super computer. NASA computers are not as efficient as the human brain.

Science still can't figure out all that the brain is capable of doing even to this date.

"Example sheds a gentle hope in which others borrow, so first improve and develop yourself today, and then your friends tomorrow." (Jeff Trigo, D.C.)

As nerves infiltrate all areas of the body what needs to be remembered is the choking compression that takes place with dislodged vertebrae. The information highway is all jammed up with traffic and the destination is greatly compromised. In other words the IVF narrowing caused by every single subluxation affects all functions and destinations of that vital nerve highway. One subluxation, defined in chapter 3, can affect organs, tissues, cells, glands, bones, muscles, skin, and more. Subluxations often remain unchecked therefore fooling most health care providers. In fact the diagnosis rendered is usually a symptom description without identifying the cause or origin in most cases. Examples: tendonitis, bursitis, sprain strain, etc. All of these diagnostic determinations may be true but yet can there be more to it?

Is it possible that vertebral subluxation complex (VSC) is present and left undetected? In most cases, the answer is yes, and VSC can cause so many unwanted symptoms and dis/ease. Life produces subluxations therefore I challenge you to view the body as an intelligent design and therefore stop trying to pop a magic pill, potion, or lotion, but instead go get your power turned on, a.k.a. adjustment and experience maximum life again. This is the expression of neuro-impulses unimpaired flowing above down from the inside out due to that gentle accurate adjustment to fine tune function and remove cause.

To take in a new idea you must destroy the old, let go of old opinions, to observe and conceive new thoughts. To learn is but to change your mind. (B. J. Palmer, DC)

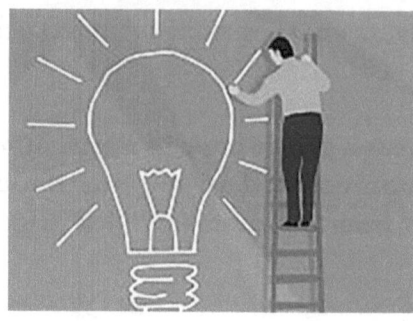

There is a paradigm shift taking place in today's world. Technology is always available with our smart phones, voice command, or asks Siri, Google, Alexa, etc., or just a webpage click away. People are learning through social media faster than ever before and knowledge can't be kept a secret any longer. People are realizing that pill popping just doesn't make sense or bring the great results desired and just totally seems like "quackery." My patients are starting to think more and more about their friend's spines when they discover for themselves how the spine is related to all functions of the human body. If someone you know or love has symptom(s), ask them if they have tried chiropractic yet? If they get resistance they don't quit, they are ninjas in patient recruitment and don't settle for that common misnomer or whatever that excuse they may have for rejecting spinal care. Instead they stay persistent because they truly care about this ailing loved one, they tell their wellness story and win the heart of the next future patient based on their own testimonials. Another life gets saved. That is why I am a chiropractor. I remove the interference that renders healing by taking away causation and then get out of the way, because patients love to heal themselves!

Without our vital connection in place, the healing pathways would be impossible. Stomachs would create too much or not enough acid. Hormone regulation would be out the window, can you imagine what kind of life we would live in without proper hormone regulation. Pipes would not have proper peristalsis (snake like movement squeezing out its contents) so they would be leaky, or bursting within us. In other words, there is way too much disease and symptoms to mention here.

As nerves exit every level of the spine, these vital connections and neuro-communication highways travel everywhere. They must be operating at 100 percent function, 100 percent of the time to maximize function and greatness within.

**"Natural forces within us are the true
healers of disease." (Hippocrates)**

With the adjustment, life is returned to normal, communication pathways return to optimal levels thus curing all sorts of ailments. If you want to really experience all that life has to offer, then stop operating with so many of your spinal circuit breakers in the off position! To get a fresh start towards wellness, one must start the correction of VSC to restore, reconnect and rejuvenate. This causes your vital nerves to operate at full power, speed and intent. Absent of traffic congestion and distortion that plagues the millions everywhere. To Heal the Nation we must restore our vital communication so that innate wisdom may operate unimpaired. VSC can rob and destroy you of your health, and can potentially cause death. Don't be fooled by its many symptoms, get adjusted instead.

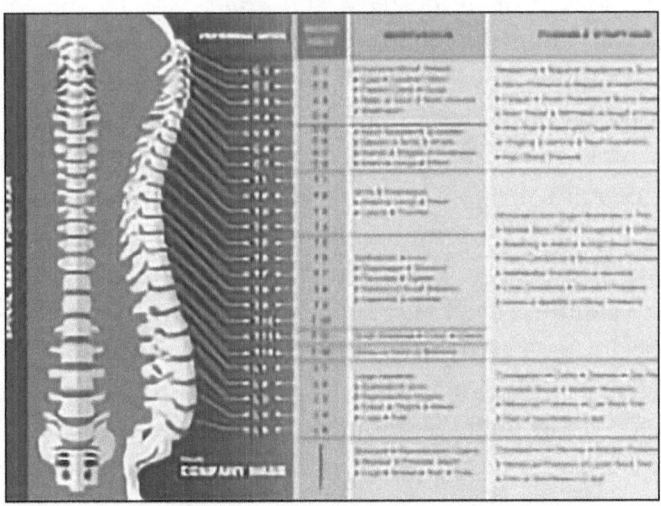

Nerve distribution to organs, tissues, glands etc.

CHAPTER 3

The Silent Killer

There is a very good reason that principled chiropractors use this term, "silent killer" when referring to the widely unknown condition in which all people are plagued with and it's called SUBLUXATION. I will discuss in a later chapter what "principled" means, but let's get back to this "silent killer," which plagues all vertebrates.

The term in Latin translates as *sub*, meaning "below the surface"; *lux*, "locked or dislocated"; and *ation*, "the act thereof." It's a very common condition that affects various joints. This locked or subluxated joint is now in a pathophysiological position and dislocated. In other words they are no long freely moveable, a.k.a. stuck, jammed, or fixated, etc. The loss of normal joint motion spells a certain doom to the joint space and nerves that exit this region. Movement is life to the joint therefore without it you can now expect the disc, cartilage, nerve size, even the shape of the bone to all have been given a diminished life span; introducing the onset of a lowered state of health such as arthritis and dis/ease, all caused by VSC.

Imagine bending your elbow to ninety degrees and putting a cast on a healthy elbow joint. Six months has passed, you take off the cast, do you think that you can freely move your elbow joint now? No way! The six-month loss of normal motion has caused muscles to atrophy and weaken. This dry elbow joint now has "arthritis," and is semi frozen. The tendon and ligament's integrity are compromised as well as the infiltration of pain with movement, etc. That was only six months; imagine fifteen to twenty-five years of having a locked spinal joint. Along with degenerative disc and joint diseases you also get organ, tissue, cells, glands, muscle and skin regions that suffer from less function, worsened mobility and loss of wellness as the subluxations effects creep in. Just like not brushing your teeth, over time the neglect will show itself.

There is a word I want you to learn and it's called imbibition, meaning to drink and/or the absorption of a liquid. This term imbibition is applied to the process of movement in which cerebral spinal fluid (CSF) is moved in and out of the joint space, bringing in oxygen rich fluid and removing the low oxygen metabolic waste out of the joint space. Without movement, the joint space rots away and becomes very arthritic and over time this premature aging is even visible on X-rays.

In the *Journal of the Neurobiological Review 2007,* leading researchers discovered that the brain is like a battery and it needs to be charged. That charge happens with normal movement of the joints. That motion sends a charge up to the brain making it a better functioning power plant, so to say, and it is able to communicate with a higher potential when properly charged. Have you ever been super tired but then got up and moved around a bit, notice how it definitely woke you right up. It is important to engage in regular exercise and plenty of movement throughout the day so that we can operate with a completely charged battery/brain. How sweet our sleep becomes when we really exerted ourselves that day.

"The sleep of a laboring man is sweet, Whether he eats little or much; But the abundance of the rich will not permit him to sleep." (Ecclesiastes 5:12)

"If we could give every individual the right amount of nourishment and exercise, not too little and not too much, we would have found the safest way to health." (Hippocrates)

What's worse than the loss of joint motion caused by the subluxation? A crushed nerve; diminishing our inner healer's message. This silent killer creates a lowered impulse that alters and diminishes neuro intent robbing you of wellness. This causes a weakening of the message that is traveling from the brain above, then down the spine and from the inside out travels that nerve pathway. With subluxation and its nerve crushing effects, our connection to life's very function has been altered and diminished. Expect symptoms and chaos as this diminishes the nerves information highway and impairs function leading to dysfunction.

The crushing pressure on a nerve will shrink the nerves diameter. I often express this using an analogy with my patients and compare it to the different sizes of pastas. Linguini becomes spaghetti in size and eventually angel hair. You will not have the same neuro-electrical impulse traveling through a smaller crushed nerve that has atrophied; now dis/ease is starting to show its ugly self.

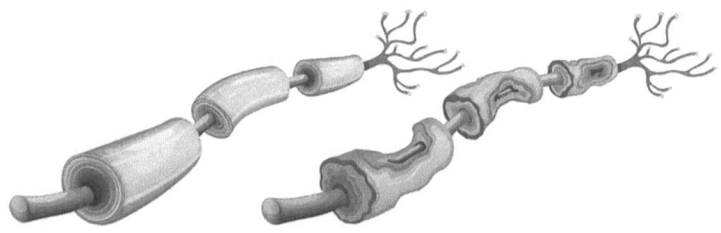

**"To comprise with anything medical in legislation
is to accept something short of full freedom which
would be part slavery." (B. J. Palmer, DC)**

There are five key components to the silent killer, a.k.a. subluxation. The spinal joint that was forced into a locked position now undergoes these dangerous pathological changes throughout the body:

1. **Kinesiopathology** (joint damage)
   Misaligned and locked spinal vertebra
   Postural imbalances, forward head carriage, a high shoulder, or low hip, etc.
   Disc stress, tears, herniation's, bulges, degenerative joint disease (DJD)
   Reduced range of motion, short or long leg, and pain

2. **Neuropathology** (nerve damage)
   Pinched, compressed, or stretched nerves
   Lower innate life flow with distortion and mixed signals
   Altered function wherever the nerve travels
   Loss of fine motor skills and power, numbness or pain

3. **Histopathology** (tissue damage)
   Inflammation, redness, heat, lactic acid accumulation, swelling, tenderness and painful to touch soft tissue areas. Premature aging, with wear and tear evident, loss of normal tissue function. Arthritic changes at effected areas. Change in bony appearance.

4. **Myopathology** (muscle damage)
   Tight muscle, guarding, or spasms in muscles. Trigger points and tightness.
   Weakness or atrophy (shrinking) in the muscle, tendon or ligament regions. Achy or sharp-stabbing, throbbing, twitching muscles, loss of sensation.
   Chronic fatigue with normal everyday stuff. Postural distortions and biomechanical improprieties are apparent, altered gait and/or pain.

5. **Pathophysiology** (health deterioration)
   Dis/ease, disc degeneration, organ malfunction, chronic illness and fatigue, loss in height with accelerated aging. Bony changes like spurs, loss of disc height and stenosis (narrowing of the IVF). Deteriorating of the compressed nerves with a failure to thrive and overall poor expression of health.

"If someone wishes for good health, one must first ask oneself if he is ready to do away with the reason for his illness. Only then is it possible to help him." (Hippocrates)

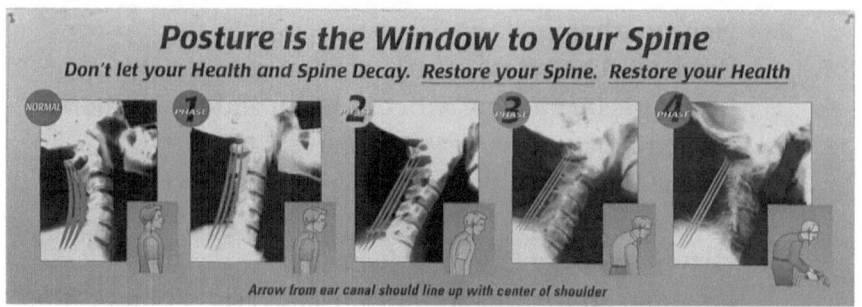

Posture is the Window to Your Spine
Don't let your Health and Spine Decay. Restore your Spine. Restore your Health

Arrow from ear canal should line up with center of shoulder

"Innate wisdom must freely flow unimpaired in order to live a life at its maximum expression." (Jeff Trigo, D.C.)

The dislocated bone, subluxation, is often referred to as vertebral subluxation complex (VSC) for short. The reason it is so complex is due to the fact that it involves a pair of spinal nerves, a disc and two vertebral bones. VSC wreaks havoc upon a lot of different regions of the body therefore leading to many unwanted symptoms and fooling most doctors into chasing the symptom instead of locating and fixing the cause. This silent killer plagues every vertebrate on the planet! News flash, the spine is no great mystery; it works like a circuit breaker.

"Educate don't medicate." (Jeff Trigo, DC)

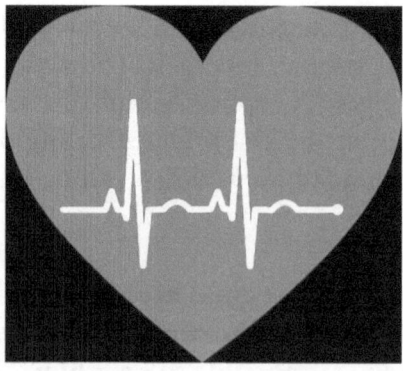

The BIG Idea

A slip on the snowy sidewalk in winter is a SMALL thing. It happens to millions.

A fall from a ladder in the summer is a SMALL thing. It also happens to millions.

The slip or fall produces a subluxation. The subluxation is a SMALL thing.

The subluxation produces pressure on a nerve. That pressure is a SMALL thing.

That decreased flowing produces a dis-eased body and brain. That is a BIG thing to that man.

Multiply that sick man by a thousand, and you control the physical and mental welfare of a city.

Multiply that man by one hundred thirty million, and you forecast and can prophesy the physical and mental status of a nation.

So the slip or fall, the subluxation, pressure, flow of mental images, and dis-ease are big enough to control the thoughts and actions of a nation.

Now comes a man. And one man is a SMALL thing.

This man gives an adjustment. The adjustment is a SMALL thing.

The adjustment replaces the subluxation. That is a SMALL thing.

The adjusted subluxation releases pressure upon nerves. That is a SMALL thing.

The released pressure restores health to a man. This is a BIG thing to that man.

Multiply that well man by a thousand, and you step up the physical and mental welfare of a city.

Multiply that well man by a million, and you increase the efficiency of a state.

Multiply that well man by a hundred thirty million, and you have produced a healthy, wealthy, and better race for posterity.

So the adjustment of the subluxation to release pressure upon nerves, to restore mental impulse flow, to restore health, is big enough to rebuild the thoughts and actions of the world.

The idea that knows the cause, that can correct the cause of dis-ease, is one of the biggest ideas known. Without it, nations fall; with it, nations rise.

This idea is the biggest I know of.

(B. J. Palmer, **1944**)

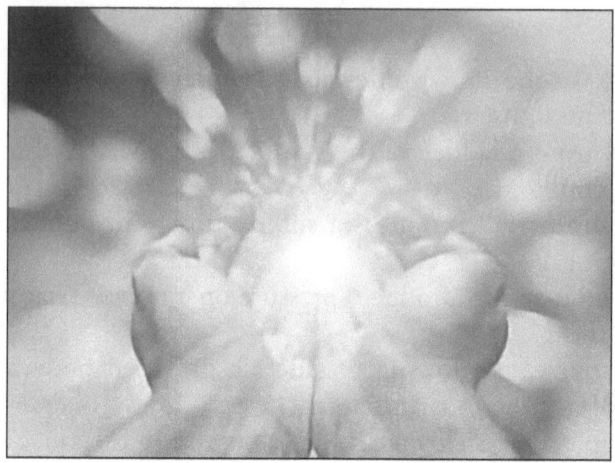

Chiropractors are the only doctors that are fully trained at finding and fixing subluxations. Would you trust your dentist to work on your feet or your ophthalmologist to do an ear exam? Then why would anyone let their massage therapist, acupuncturist, or medical doctor manipulate their spine? I used the term manipulation for a reason. Chiropractors adjust! When I use the term *manipulation*, I am referring to a nonspecific movement on a region that uses high force and low speed and a long lever. An example of this would be someone that is lying on their side and the person giving the manipulation is contacting the patients shoulder and leg while twisting and it's very possible that many bones will articulate, "Pop." On the contrary, when an adjustment is given, there is one specific targeted vertebra or joint that will move. The patient will not hear multiple popping sounds like in a manipulation. The chiropractor uses a short lever, high speed and low force technique that will adjust and correct all xyz vectors of the subluxation.

1. The anterior-posterior vector of the subluxation
2. The rotational vector of the subluxation
3. The superior-inferior wedging vector of the subluxation

An example of precision adjustment would be a patient laying on their side, and the doctor places his hand on the vertebra that is tender to the touch, subluxated, and moves only that bone in a specific vector, direction to correct (VSC). He determined the vector by careful spinal palpation techniques, motion testing each joint segment and if needed confirming via diagnostic methods like X-ray, MRI, etc.

Failure to get your spine checked on a regular basis is wellness sabotage. Consider this, all subluxation turn into a degenerative state of existence. Would you ever consider avoiding teeth brushing for months or years? That sounds absurd right, well you can get a new tooth but you can't get a new spine. Your spine will rot away just like teeth do and yet chiropractors have done a poor job with educating the public on this versus the dentist whom have knocked it out of the entire ball park with their education Home Run on cavity prevention and daily brushing and flossing importance. Why do chiropractors only see 10 percent of the population?

If the chiropractor would take the time on every new patient and teach them how, no matter what we do, our freely moveable spine can and will move into a locked position, and that we all get subluxations, then maybe this message can go viral. When undetected there are too many symptoms to list here that will absolutely creep into the unwanted self therefore loss of wellness is eminent without chiropractic maintenance. It takes a bit of time to teach the patient that the progression of the untreated subluxation rots the spine away causing dis/ease and loss of life. Set a standard of frequency that will be best for the patient with no gap in care that exceeds two weeks. It has been seen on a MRI that a hydrated disc is whiter than the dehydrated and degenerated disc, which disseminates and turns gray. It has been documented that when a subluxation occurs, the white disc starts to turn gray within two weeks on MRI. Discs have a great capacity to hold water at a ratio of 17:1. These shock absorbing sponges can dry up with loss of fluid flow. Have you ever tried to bend a dried up sponge? It cracks and tears just like the human disc that has lost its imbibition ability. Adjustments are paramount for life.

Hierarchy of Life

This is the order of small parts making up larger parts eventually becoming our human design. So when you see a word above, just add many more of them and they become the next word below.

Atom
Molecule
Macromolecule
Organelle
Cell: the first unit of life
Tissue
Organ
System
Human

When given a medication to change the body's function, what level does this drug interact with? If you said cellular level you are correct. Now with an adjustment, this affects a much higher level of structures closer to the human level, skeletal system/nervous system, hence obtaining much faster and safer results. So trying to change the function at the cellular level to help alter tissues to affect organs and eventually work its way into systems like cardiovascular or immune, digestive, muscular systems, etc., to affect the human function is ludicrous. Chiropractors adjust bones off nerves to affect systems and the results are faster and safer absent of playing pill-popping Russian roulette with your biochemistry. Pills will change your cellular function and trigger them to do something that is altered and unnatural. MDs hand out prescription pills like Halloween candy. Why are chiropractors only adjusting 10 percent of the population? We need to ramp up our marketing strategies to save more lives! Only skilled Chiropractors adjust by hand and remove the cause of the symptom at the source, VSC.

If people would first get checked for (VSC), the world would still have many of its stars, less disabilities, there would be less drug addiction to pills, opioids, etc., and life would absolutely be fun again as you live a pain free life with pep to your step.

The sooner that people realize, that no matter what they do, our spines will get subluxated sooner or later. All life long, on everybody, guaranteed 100 percent. Same is true that everybody needs to brush their teeth; well, everybody needs to stay adjusted. You may be asking by now, I wonder if I have a subluxation? Well, let me say this, you were all born and that's where most traumas begin. Then by the time you learned to walk before the age of two you fell approximately 1,500 times. Add gravity, poor posture, sports traumas, sleeping in a bad positions, lifting wrong, car accidents, repetitive traumas, emotional, physical and chemical stressors. Our spine is being exposed to all kinds of forces at multiple levels, often experiencing multiple levels of subluxation and therefore fooling most doctors because they are not looking for the cause but again chasing symptoms with pill-popping, horrendous overprescribing habits. Shift your thought patterns, first check the circuit breaker before the pills, scalpel or bolt. Odds are that a subluxation exists pinching a nerve and that dimmer switch on function is expressing its loss of innate wisdom and being with symptoms means you are not living at life's highest potential, thus loss of wellness! You don't only brush your teeth when you have a cavity, do you? If so, you don't get the regular brushing benefit. Same is true for chiropractic. I don't want my patients only coming in when they are sick, have a headache, or are experiencing sciatica or that one thing or another. Instead I want them coming in for maintenance of wellness. Absent of dis/ease and symptoms, also absent of a sickness story.

If you are in a health crisis, my hopes are that you get out of pain ASAP and begin a series of spinal correction adjustments to fix subluxations and the postural deficits. Address any toxicities and deficiencies—include habits of great nutrition and exercise. These are all future chapters to look forward to. Adjustments are safe hence very desirable results are obtained while being very cost effective at the same time. God uses chiropractors to heal His people!

"An ounce of prevention is worth a pound of cure." (Benjamin Franklin)

Don't let past traumas, slips and falls rob you of your health. All spines are exposed to thousands of forces over the course of our lifetime that are capable of causing vertebral subluxation complex, VSC for short!

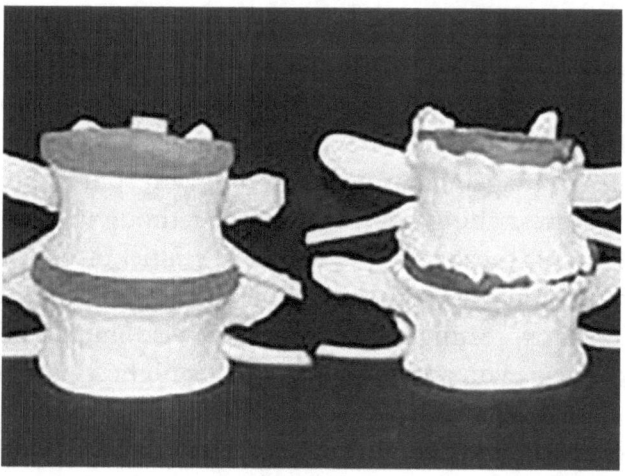

The vertebra on the left is normal, square in shape, and without arthritis. The disc have remained lubricated and the pair of spinal nerves that exit are working at the highest potential possible. The vertebra on the right has been locked for at least 10-15 years, it's degenerative, spurs are visible, there is now spinal stenosis, nerve atrophy is the byproduct thereof and dis/ease is evident. Adjustments add years to your life and life to your years. If you want to age to perfection, it's definitely a choice! I choose to Get Adjusted!

CHAPTER 4

Toxicities and Deficiencies

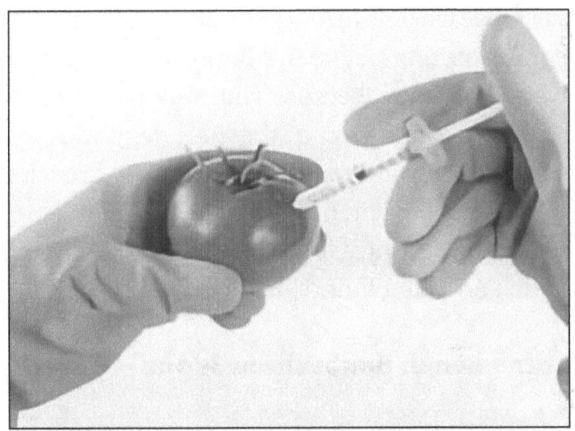

Having the mind-set that our body is brilliantly and divinely designed and with a life span of 120 years according to the Bible of the post-flood man, then a more logical way of reasoning might be to consider these two questions when loss of wellness becomes expressive. Consider this:

1. Is there anything toxic in your body? If so, remove it at the source.
2. Is there a deficiency present? Add it exactly as needed in all circumstances.

By answering these questions above, we can definitely approach healthcare differently than what is mainstream today. This yields different results that are more desirable than the endless prescription drugs and surgical approach. After all most people view our healthcare system as broken, bankrupt and failed. I hope to shift the way the public views symptoms and learns the many alternative natural remedies available that are holistic and safe. So consider these concepts as you read on.

We, as a society, do not have a system in place in which the people of the nation can get educated and learn about life promoting foods. Where is the class or nutritional program that teaches the general public how to read labels? To be able to understand useful fats versus the bad fats, good and bad sugars, etc. It's just not taught. Therefore take responsibility upon yourself to learn as much as you can about toxic products being offered to the unsuspecting public. It's important to know what you are putting in or on your body, because you only have one. This chapter should make it easy to know a few of the most dangerous most common ingredients to avoid. You will also learn common deficiencies that lead to illness. You can use this book as a quick reference guide for many health benefits while promoting longevity without risky side effects and adverse drug reactions that are often found via modern medicine.

"Remember when in doubt throw it out" (Jeff Trigo, DC)

Try to keep the number of combined ingredients to a maximum of five and let them be words you can pronounce; naturally existing in nature and not processed in a factory or laboratory. Have your food be free from food coloring, dyes, preservatives and not from the frozen section. This real food can be found in the outer perimeter of the grocery stores, not in the center isles. Organic is best, free of pesticides and sprays. This means you may have to shop more often to keep fresh organic produce on your kitchen tables. And buy locally grown, this lowers the carbon footprint on the environment.

"We all have big changes in our lives that are more or less a second chance." (Harrison Ford)

48

A well-balanced diet that is packed with naturally dense nutrients is essential to a healthy life. Grown organically and in soil that has not been depleted of its strength to grow dark colored fruits and vegetables; soil rich in vitamins and minerals! If you keep in mind that health is accumulative, then creating wholesome eating habits is essential toward wellness.

Malnutrition and deficiencies due to a loss of the well-balanced diet that is lacking in some of the essential elements can lead to these common diseases:

Beri Beri: Vitamin B1 deficiency. It's an illness that alters muscle function, nerve degeneration, and cardiovascular problems. B1, also known as thiamine, can be found in beef, beans, eggs, whole oats and grains, nuts, oranges and pork.

Depression: Vitamin B7 deficiency. Mental issues, hair loss, skin disorders, dry eyes, dry or scaly skin, loss of appetite, sleep loss, insomnia. B7 also known as Biotin can be found in liver, corn, egg yolks, wheat brand, avocados, broccoli, cauliflower, cheese, mushrooms, nuts potatoes, spinach, dark leafy greens, beans, fish, chicken, pork and dairy products. Also check for C1–2 subluxations.

Goiter: Iodine deficiency, causing the thyroid gland to enlarge leading to hypothyroidism, poor growth, hindrances for proper childhood development, cretinism, always cold, changes in heart rate, weight gain, fatigue, hair loss, and learning disabilities. Iodine can be found in enriched salts, fish especially cod, shrimp and tuna, eggs, seaweed, Kombu kelp, dairy, prunes, and lima beans. Check C7 vertebra, misalignments will crush the nerves that go to the thyroid gland.

Iron Deficiency Anemia: Iron deficiency, causing a decrease in red blood cells or hemoglobin in the body thus reducing the body's oxygen carrying capabilities resulting in fatigue, weakness, paleness, and dyspnea. Foods rich in iron include squashes, tofu, nuts, spinach, lentil, dark chocolate, broccoli, raisins, navy beans, chickpeas, oysters, quinoa, beef, turkey, fish, liver, pumpkin seed, cashews, potatoes, split peas, kidney beans, red meat, and figs.

"Eat to live don't live to eat." (Benjamin Franklin)

Kwashiorkor: A protein deficiency in the body that is caused by malnutrition and starvation. The enlarged liver gives the appearance of an extended abdomen; Anorexic child with a pregnancy look. Rust looking skin, loss of muscle mass, failure to grow, fatigue, swelling ankles feet and belly, diarrhea, frequent infections and irritability. Diet lacks proteins found in meats, eggs, fish, beans, and nuts.

Osteoporosis: Vitamin D and calcium deficiency in the body therefore weakening the boney matrix of the skeletal system. As bone becomes less dense, pathological compression fractures of the spine are common and/or hip fractures, etc. Sources of calcium include wild fatty fish (tuna, mackerel, and salmon), cheese, egg yolks, and beef, liver, orange juice, almond milk, fortified dairy products, shiitake mushrooms, and oatmeal.

Pellagra: Vitamin B3 (niacin) deficiency. Characteristics include the four Ds: diarrhea, dementia, dermatitis, and death. The disease is also accompanied by a loss of the amino acids tryptophan and lysine. Heavy levels of lysine will cause the four D's. Foods rich in niacin are tuna, whole grains, mushrooms, peanuts, chicken, green peas, and liver.

Rickets: Vitamin D deficiency along with poor absorption of calcium and potassium. The result of this deficiency leads to soft and weak bones, bowed legs, short stature, deformed bones and teeth, muscle cramps, and fractures. Treatment includes increased exposure to sunlight, consumption of fatty fish, liver, milk, eggs, cheese, orange juice, soy, and other fortified products like dairy.

Scurvy: Vitamin C (ascorbic acid) deficiency. This disease inhibits the formation of collagen production in the body which is the structural protein in connective tissue. Symptoms include, skin sores, scabs, decaying gums, abnormal appearance of teeth and bones. Poor wound healing and bleeding gums. Treatment is to make sure your diet is packed with fresh fruits like lemons, limes, oranges, strawberries, broccoli, Brussel sprouts, kiwi, papaya, cantaloupe, bell peppers, tomatoes, grapefruit, and kale.

Xerophthalmia: Also known as night blindness a.k.a. nyctalopia caused by vitamin A deficiency. One of the early symptoms is the inability to produce tears. The deficiency impairs immunity, affects the ocular region. This is due to an impairment of dark adaptation due to lack of photoreceptor pigment rhodopsin. Xerophthalmia: dry thickening of the conjunctiva and cornea. Bitot spots: Keratinized growth (metaplasia) on the conjunctiva causing hazy vision. Treatment: consumptions of carrots, sweet potatoes, green leafy vegetables, cantaloupe, fish, pumpkin, liver, parsley, and meat.

Vitamins should be carefully considered when going to the store to purchase. First off, they must be water soluble. When put in a glass of water, the supplement should have no problem dissolving. I know very popular brands of vitamins that are peddled to the un-expecting public that won't dissolve and you can even see it on X-ray as it moves through the large intestines. In other words you're flushing your money down the drain. I have always liked plant based natural greens and whole food supplements over any chemically manufactured substance or pill. Look for natural safe and 100 percent bio-dissolvable supplements. A separate multi-mineral that is also plant based is suggested and other supplements based on age, eating habits, weight goals, etc. This will be discussed more in depth in later chapters. Remember that a vitamin is a catalyst that speeds up the metabolic process. It's almost impossible to eat the perfect well-balanced diet that has no deficiencies or toxicities, therefore supplementation should be considered to give your body what it needs. Most soils have been depleted of its natural nutrients to grow rich vibrant foods high in the vitamins, minerals, and fibers, etc. These elements are beneficial to our health. The reason we are in a poor soil zone is due to the fact that we did not take heed the divine instructions in regards ancient day composting:

Six years you shall sow your field, and six years you shall prune your vineyard, and gather its fruit; but in the seventh year there shall be a Sabbath of solemn rest for the land a Sabbath to the LORD. You shall neither sow your fields nor prune your vineyard. What grows of its own accord of your harvest you shall not reap, nor gather the grapes of your untended vine, for it is a year of rest for the land. (Leviticus 5:3–5)

The season's harvest of fruits and vegetables will all fall to the ground, decompose and enrich the soil giving back that which was depleted. Today we mostly compost to feed our trees and replenish our soil; it's organic and natural while being effective for growing nutrient dense foods.

"Subluxation is a major deficiency in joint motion and nerve supply therefore fooling most doctors into chasing the symptom instead of locating the cause." (Jeff Trigo, DC)

Any lack or too much of the following can lead to serious health issues so here is another useful list of Vitamins and Minerals that are needed for a healthy lifestyle. I will include some common foods that are naturally high in these supplements, so that one could make the necessary diet changes for better nutritional balance.

Remember when buying natural supplements, look for labels that represent doses as close to 100 percent of the recommended daily allowance needed to maximize optimal function and reduce the chance of deficiencies and toxicities. When possible, eat a variety of organically grown fruits and vegetables as a preference over taking supplements.

"Let medicine be thy food and food be thy medicine." (Hippocrates)

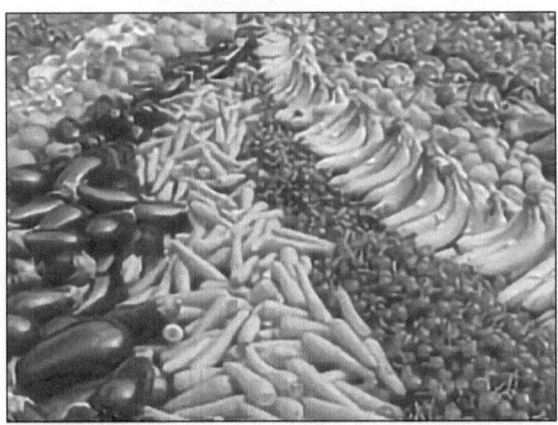

Vitamin A: The leading cause of preventable blindness in children and lack of it causes disease and death. In pregnancy a deficiency can lead to maternal mortality. Vitamin A is an essential nutrient and is particularly good for vision, skin acne, reproductive health, immunity, body growth and hair.

Sources: Liver, fish, cheese, eggs, sweet potato, winter squash, kale, collards, turnip greens, carrots, sweet red peppers, Swiss chard, spinach, romaine lettuce, mango, cantaloupe, grape fruit, watermelon apricot, papaya, tangerine, passion fruit, guava, and nectarine.

RDA: 5000 IU

B vitamins: They all mostly aid in nervous system function as well as metabolism and energy. In general they are mostly found in fish, meats, and green leafy veggies. Toxic levels of B vitamins causes polyneuropathies = many nerve pains.

Vitamin B1 Thiamin: Helps the body's cells convert carbohydrates into energy that is used especially for brain and nerve conduction; aids in muscle contraction. A lack of B1 can lead to beri beri and causes weakness, fatigue, psychosis, GI problems, muscle and nerve damage. Alcohol robs your body of B1.

Sources: Soy beans, peas, enriched grains and cereals, nuts, pork, seeds, liver, oats, oranges, fish, pumpkin squash, cooked asparagus and enriched breads.

RDA: 1.5mg

> **"Good nutrition creates health in all areas of our existence. All parts are interconnected." (T. Collin Campbell)**

Vitamin B2 Riboflavin: Important for healthy skin, eyes and nervous system function. Aids in metabolism, energy production from the food we eat. If our body is low in this vitamin we see cracks in the corner of the mouth, angular stomatitis. We also observe cracks on the tongue, glossitis, corneal vascularization, red scaly skin inflammations, greasy patches on the eyelids, nose, scrotum, and labia, and some types of anemias.

Sources: Eggs, mushrooms, meat, cheese, milk, almonds, spinach, nuts, liver, fish, yogurt, green leafy vegetables, wholegrains, soybeans, and broccoli.

RDA: 1.7mg

Vitamin B3 Niacin: Important for continued nerve function and metabolism, a common theme amongst all B vitamins, as well as healthy skin. Toxicity of niacin has been known to damage the liver, causes depression, disorientation, and possibly nausea and/or vomiting.

Sources: Chicken, fish, pork, beef, nuts, beans, seafood, green leafy vegetables, mushrooms, brown rice, avocados, and sweet potatoes.

RDA: 20mg

> **"The best time to start eating well is from birth. The second best time is right now!" (Jeff Trigo, DC)**

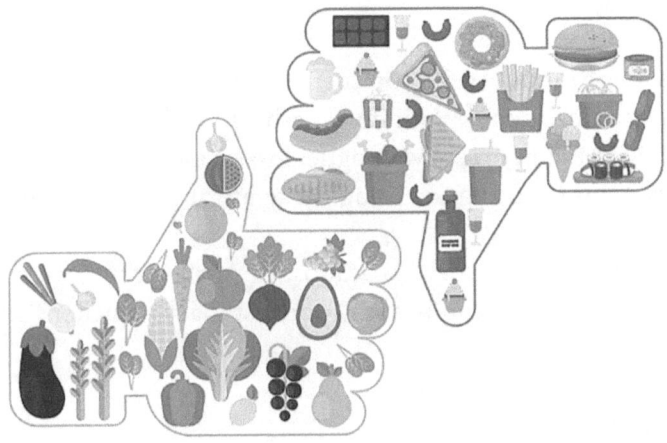

"Healing is a matter of time but it is sometimes also a matter of opportunity." (Hippocrates)

Vitamin B5 Pantothenic Acid: B5 helps regulate metabolism, nerve conduction and function. Therefore if one has low levels of B5 you may see low energy levels, a fatigued stressed and depressed state of condition, anxiety, etc.

Sources: Chicken, eggs, fish, pork, beef, nuts, beans, seafood, green leafy vegetables, mushrooms, avocados, brown rice, sweet potatoes, and yogurts.

RDA: 10mg

Vitamin B6 Pyridoxine: A water soluble vitamin that aids in metabolism, proper red blood cell (RBC's) production, as well as nervous system and immune system optimization. Deficiencies lead to skin disorders, energy loss, depression, fatigue, anxiety, confusion, convulsions, and anemias.

Sources: Pork, beef, chicken, salmon, sweet potatoes, bananas, avocados, nuts especially pistachios.

RDA: 1.7mg

Vitamin B7 Biotin: An important substance for the metabolism of fat. Deficiencies include hair loss, rash around the nose, face and genitals, depression, excessive fatigue, loss of balance, hallucinations, numbness, and shooting neurological symptoms into legs and arms.

Sources: Organ meats, fish, avocados, egg yolks, corn, mushrooms, beans, nuts, broccoli, cauliflower, pork, spinach, chicken, fish, and potatoes.

RDA: Adult 30mcg

"Exercise is King. Nutrition is Queen. Put them together and you've got a Kingdom." (Jack LaLanne)

Vitamin B9 Folate: Helps form healthy RBCs, important for DNA synthesis, cell growth, division and repair and is important for proper fetal development. Deficiencies can lead to low blood volume = anemias, fatigue, weakness, pale skin, lethargy = without strength. Low levels also cause irritability, weight loss, spinal abnormalities, shortness of breath, gray hair, tongue swelling, heart palpitations, and mouth sores.

Sources: Asparagus, avocados, broccoli, edamame, lentils, lettuce, mangos, and oranges.

RDA: 400mcg

Vitamin B12 Cobalamin: Deficiencies are primarily symptomatic in the small intestines; Crohn's and Celiac disease, gastritis, etc. Anemia is common because B12 helps in the production of RBC's, so lower RBC counts, fatigue, fast heart rate (tachycardia). Poly-neuropathies, memory loss, bad moods, comprehension compromise, stomach lining thins, and tongue swelling

Sources: Animal liver and kidneys, clams, fish, dairy, eggs, and cheese.

RDA: 2.4mcg

Vitamin C Ascorbic acid: Deficiency in C is linked to the famous disease sailors would get when citrus was not accessible on sea called Scurvy. Poor wound healing, scaly skin and red dots with open wounds that don't heal. Gum disease, a.k.a. gingivitis. They also were labeled as "Limeys" because they would set sail with limes on board to prevent this disease. The reason for the skin lesions is due to the body's inability to make collagen when C is deficient. C is an important antioxidant, works with the immune system for better function too.

Sources: Lemons, limes, tangerines, kumquats, oranges, strawberries, kiwifruit, dragon fruit, lychees, tomatoes, peppers, cantaloupe, broccoli, Brussel sprouts, kale, spinach, cauliflower, guavas, papayas, black currants, cherries, plums, parsley, thyme, persimmons, and rose hips.

RDA: 60mg

Vitamin D: One of the most common deficiencies found today. It's a very important vitamin for blood pressure regulation, calcium absorption, balance, immune system function, bone growth, hormone production, and nervous system function. Deficiencies include these possible symptoms: weakened immune system, fatigue, weak bones that may easily fracture especially in the elderly, depression, body aches, poor wound healing, and hair loss.

Sources: Fatty fish like tuna, mackerel and salmon, cheese, egg yolks, and fortified dairy products. We must also include exposure to sunlight, and possibly supplementation.

RDA: 400–800IU

Vitamin E: Another powerful antioxidant, Vitamin C, E also aids in immunity, RBC production and proper organ function, arterial health, and other numerous benefits like anti-aging and fights against disease.

Sources: Green leafy vegetables, seeds and nuts, avocados, wheat germ, kiwi, broccoli, peppers, mango, fish, and shellfish.
   RDA: Adult 1000–1500IU

Vitamin K: An important vitamin for blood clotting and the formation of strong healthy bones. A good supplement if aspirin has been abused. Deficiencies include excessive bleeding.

Sources: Dark green leafy vegetables, parsley, cabbage, beef, liver, pork, chicken, bacon, duck, kiwi, cheese, avocadoes, egg yolks, berries, figs, tomatoes, pomegranate, nuts, and kidney beans.

RDA: 80–120mcg

Vitamins and minerals are essential nutrients in our body. Acting in unison they are performing tasks by the hundreds; healing wounds, building up our bone storage and density, aiding in immune system function, cellular repair and speeding up the process like a catalyst turning food into usable energy for our body while keeping us warm.

Minerals are very important in our overall health. Every time our heart beats it's using minerals for that important muscle to contract and relax. Minerals can be stored in our skeletal system up to the age of approximately forty. After forty we start taking these stored up minerals out of our bone. This is due to the hormonal changes we see in the blood stream at that age. It is very important to make sure that your mineral "bank deposit" is large by the age of forty. Minerals also aid in transmitting nerve impulses, hormone production and help you grow.

"When diet is wrong, medicine is of no use. When diet is correct medicine is of no need." (Ancient Ayurveda Proverb)

Mineral deficiencies are a common problem today. Many people are low in these vital elements and are susceptible to cramps, eye twitching, fatigue, illness and injury that could have be prevented. Before I give you a list of minerals, the role they play in the importance of our health and their natural sources, I thought I should let you know of the everyday foods that are robbing you of your minerals.

Sugar: Found in almost everything now a days. Not found naturally on the planet but made in a laboratory when combining glucose + sucrose = table sugar. FYI: Cancer loves sugar! Primarily found in soda, candy, desserts, cereal, juice, condiments, and baked goods. It also comes in many forms: agave nectar, brown sugar, caramel, dextrose, cane crystals, cane sugar, crystalline fructose, evaporated cane juice, fructose, glucose, sucrose, honey, lactose, maltose, malt syrup, molasses, syrup. Cause of type-2 diabetes and obesity.

Sugar robs your body of: Vitamin C, calcium, and magnesium.

High-Fructose Corn Syrup: 130 percent more potent than sugar, talk about a diabetic overload! It's an addictive food that triggers the brain to keep eating often leading to obese conditions. Also found in corn sweeteners, corn syrup and corn sugar. Found in junk food, candies, cereals, condiments, and many other food items because it's cheap and addictive. Keep your eyes out for this harmful additive.

Robs your body of: Zinc, magnesium, and chromium

Pectin: Found in jams, jellies, fruit juices, frosting, and yogurts.

This glue like substance robs you of fibers and other vital nutrients like antioxidants, etc. Eat natural pectins like apples instead of foods with pectin additives.

Pectin robs your body of: Beta-carotene, lycopene, and lutein.

Disodium EDTA (Ethylenediaminetetraacetic Acid): Found in processed foods. It's a preservative that helps food retain color and flavors, however it pulls metals both good and bad from the gut, leaving you with an unbalanced bacteria level that is unhealthy for proper digestive function.

EDTA robs your body of: Vitamin C, magnesium, calcium, potassium, iron, and zinc.

Phosphoric Acid: A chemical additive that keeps carbonated drinks from going flat. This additive robs your body of vital minerals needed for healthy bones.

Phosphoric acid robs your body of: Calcium, magnesium.

Guar Gum: This fiber functions as a thickener and feeds gut bacteria which robs the body of its vital elements to thrive.

Guar gum robs your body of: Beta-carotene, lycopene, and lutein.

Synthetic Sulfites: Also called Sodium sulfites, sulfur dioxide, calcium sulfites, and sodium disulfide. Commonly found in potatoes, shrimp, wine, beer and white rice.

Robs your body of: Thiamine B1

"The food you eat can be the most powerful form of medicine or the slowest form of poison." (Ann Wigmore)

Minerals

Calcium: Important in bone and teeth formation, muscle contractions, proper nervous system function, hormone secretion, blood clotting and arterial pressure. Deficiencies cause cramps, weak bones, too much causes kidney stones, and constipation.

Sources: Dairy, nuts, seeds, coconuts, green leafy vegetables, cabbage, fortified cereals and drinks, fish with bones like sardines, scallops, oysters, beans, lentils, hummus, oranges, figs, carrots, tomatoes, tahini and whole wheat.

RDA: 1000–2000mg

Chloride: Aids in blood PH acid alkaline balance (7.34 normal bodies PH). Converts food into energy/metabolism, digestive health, fluid and electrolyte balance also nervous system function.

Sources: Sea salt, pink Himalayan salt, olives, seaweed, tomatoes, rye, celery, lettuce, cabbage, cauliflower, broccoli, radish, and Brussel sprouts.

RDA: 750–900mg

Chromium: Aids diabetics in insulin function while helping metabolize proteins, fats, and carbohydrates; important for proper brain function.

Sources: Broccoli, lettuce, green beans, oats, barley, potatoes, tomatoes, apples, bananas, beef, turkey, nuts, garlic, basil, grains and egg yolks.

RDA: 50–200mcg

Copper: Helps kill free radicals (antioxidant), aids in bone formation, energy production, metabolize and works with iron to from RBCs, assures proper growth, collagen and connective tissue formation and proper nervous system function. Copper is important in immunity in making white blood cells. High levels affect GI, liver, and kidney function.

Sources: Oysters, shellfish, offal, beans, nuts, potatoes, whole grains, dark leafy greens, dried fruits, prunes, cocoa, liver, black pepper and yeast.

RDA: 1–1.6mg

Iodine: Important for proper thyroid hormone and reproductive function, growth, development and metabolism. If the levels are off it can cause a change in weight, levels too high causes weight loss, levels too low can cause weight gain.

Sources: Seaweed, Kombu kelp, nori (seaweed paper), cod, shrimp, tuna, eggs, dairy, turkey, potatoes, prunes and lima beans.

RDA: 150mcg

Iron: Important in RBC formation, energy production, growth and development, immune and reproductive system optimization, and wound healing; 70 percent of your iron is found in the blood in the form of hemoglobin and in muscle cells called myoglobin. Hemoglobin is responsible for the transfer of oxygen into the blood from the lungs. Deficiencies include anemias; toxic levels cause constipation, nausea, vomiting, and stomach pains.

Sources: Dark leafy greens, beans, beef, chicken, turkey, seafood, lamb, prunes, raisins, whole grains, broccoli, quinoa, dark chocolate, nuts, seeds, and potatoes.

RDA: 16–19mg

Magnesium: Important for bone formation, muscle contraction, blood pressure and blood sugar regulation, nervous and immune system function, aids in blood pressure and energy regulation and is involved the function of hormone secretion. Helps keep the heart rate regular and is needed for proper protein and DNA formation. Deficiencies can cause cramping and weaker bones. Toxic levels can cause diarrhea, nausea, cramping, vomiting, dizziness, and drops in blood pressure, cardio arrhythmias, and/or cardiac arrest, coma and death. Remember to take the supplements that are near or at the proper RDA.

Sources: Green leafy vegetables, avocados, bananas, nuts, seeds, beans, seafood, Brussel sprouts, quinoa, whole grains, chick peas, peanuts, and edamame.

RDA: 400mg

> **"Health is not about the weight you lose, but about the life you gain!" (Dr. Josh Axe)**

Manganese: Helps the body to absorb calcium, aids in wound healing, cartilage and bone formation, blood sugar regulation and nerve health. This mineral aids in blood clotting, sex hormone production, fat and carbohydrate metabolism. Long term consumption of too much manganese has caused muscle pain, abnormal nerve function, fatigue, and depression. Deficiencies cause poor skeletal development with week bones and deformities. Low levels also lead to the failure of collagen to be produced in wound healing, hormonal imbalance and possible infertility, anemias, fatigue and a weakened immune system.

Sources: Mussels, spinach, nuts, beans, sweet potatoes, wheat germ, chickpeas, pineapples, garlic, oats, brown rice, Quinoa, barley, rye, cloves, raspberries, corn, turmeric, kale, pumpkin seeds, green beans and Tofu.

RDA: 2mg

Phosphorus: Helps to build strong teeth and bone, an important mineral for the proper function of tissue and cell repair. Phosphorus deficiencies cause weaker bone formation, also a less dense bony matrix, a possible cause of rickets in children. It is rare to observe toxic levels, however this can lead to diarrhea, hardening of organs and skin.

Sources: Meats, chicken, seafood, dairy, beans, seeds, nuts and whole grains.

RDA: 750–1250mg

Potassium: Is an important mineral that helps nerve impulses to interact properly with muscles. The heart is a very important muscle, and this mineral aids in proper cardio rhythms and strength of contractions. Helps to maintain healthy fluid electrolyte balance and is involved with many other functions due to the fact that it can act as an electrical charge in its nerve firing action potential and blood pressure regulation. Toxic levels cause diarrhea, nausea and stomach pain. Deficiencies include weakness, fatigue, cramping, body and muscle aches, stiffness, numbness and/or tingling, heart arrhythmias, mood alterations, and GI symptoms.

Sources: Bananas, beetroot, oranges, tomatoes, potatoes, yogurt, spinach, white beans, clam, avocado, coconut, salmon, acorn squash, pomegranate juice, and watermelon.

RDA: 2500–4000mg

Selenium: Is an antioxidant, slows cellular aging, aids in metabolism and proper thyroid function. Immune and reproductive system benefits as well. Deficiency leads to possible GI and immune system compromise. Levels too high are usually from supplementation and can lead to brittle hair, loss of hair, fatigue and irritability. Toxic levels lead to stomach aches, nausea, G.I issues and halitosis, aka foul breath.

Sources: Seafood especially yellowfin tuna, chicken, eggs, meats, nuts esp. Brazilian, whole grains, dairy, bananas, mushrooms, and sunflower seeds.

RDA: 80–200 mcg

Sodium: Functions in fluid balance, acid base body Ph. balance, muscle contractions, nervous system function, blood pressure and blood volume regulation.

Sources: Salt, used as a preservative in canned soups, vegetables, condiments, meats, cheeses, pizza, fast food, fries, pretzels, chips, pickles, cold cuts, canned fish, nuts, chili, and sausage. All of these foods are high in sodium so be watchful of your daily intake. I personally suggest using the pink Himalayan salt, it's not bleached and can be found naturally in nature.

RDA: 1800–2400mg

Zinc: Important for the proper function of smell and taste. It also aids in digestion. An important mineral found in our body that functions in cell growth and cellular division, metabolizes carbohydrates, works with optimizing our immune response and reproductive system, development and growth, and nervous system function. Deficiencies include poor growth, impaired immune system, eye and skin lesions with loss of hair and appetite, poor sexual development. Toxic levels give the body abdominal cramps and indigestion, vomiting, nausea, loss of appetite, diarrhea and possible headaches.

Sources: Oysters, lobster, shrimp, crab, chicken, meat, dairy, nuts, beans, whole grains, nuts, cereal, wheat germ, avocados, berries, peas, and pomegranates.

RDA: 13mg

Something to consider: Sometimes you will find yourself at a toxic location or in a toxic relationship or even in a friendship that doesn't honor God. Remove yourself ASAP; minimizing the negative effects it will have on your peace of mind, while also reducing the amount of collateral damage on those around you. Have zero lag time here. The key to success lies in your ability for early recognition and implication of action to change.

> **"Chiropractic, like gravity, works whether you
> believe it or not." (Sid E. Williams)**

Surround yourself with people that you want to emulate, not tolerate. Strive to implement greatness in all you do. Whether it's picking your food, choosing your friends and/or where you spend your time, make sure it is good for your body, mind and soul. Consider the consequences of bad choices before you indulge in them and have an accountability partner that you check in with at least weekly to make sure you're are on purpose with your life goals. Goals to be monitored are in multiple areas of your life: financial, spiritual, relationship with others and physical.

> **"Do not be deceived, God is not mocked; for whatever
> a man sows, that he will also reap." (Galatians 6:7)**

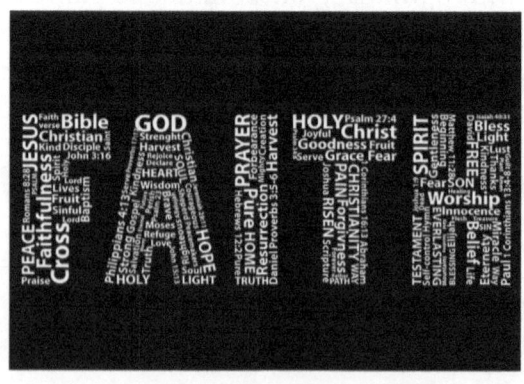

Random Toxins You Must Avoid:

Microwaveable popcorn!
BPA plastics, they are carcinogens
Artificial sweeteners
Fat-free foods
Vegetable oils, they damage arteries.
Margarine or Crisco = Trans fat
Food coloring (Blue 1 and 2, green 3, red 3, and yellow 6)
Hydrogenated oils
Bleached flour
Monosodium Glutamate (MSG) messes with brain chemistry
High-fructose corn syrup/corn syrup (130
percent more potent than sugar)
Agave
Sugar
Carrageenan (indigestible polysaccharide)
Isolated soy protein (indigestible protein)
GMO foods
Caged eggs
Farm raised and color added foods
Canned beans (cans lined With BPA)
Canned veggies (cans lined with BPA)
Shortening and other unsaturated fats including
trans fats, palm oil, mineral oil
Mammograms, the test to detect cancer is
the leading cause of breast cancer
Sodium benzoate (carcinogen in soda); potassium
benzoate (carcinogen in soda)
Aspirin leads to hemorrhage. NSAIDs lead to kidney cyst and
inhibit cartilage formation. Acetaminophen leads to kidney and
liver damage. Cortisone lowers immunity and causes increased
inflammation while reducing the mobility of Natural Killer Cells;
lowering our innate ability for fighting cancer. Opioids lead to
drug addiction, drug dependency and death due to overdose.
Butylated Hydroxyanisole (carcinogenic preservative)

Sodium nitrates and sodium nitrites (carcinogens found in bacon, hot dogs and lunch meats). Also avoid cooking with Teflon non-stick cooking pans
Smog and exhaust for those intersections as you sit with the window down, it's poison. Carbon monoxide has a two hundred times more affinity to cling on to that RBC.

"Every time you eat or drink, you are either promoting disease or combating it" (Jeff Trigo, DC)

Pesticide

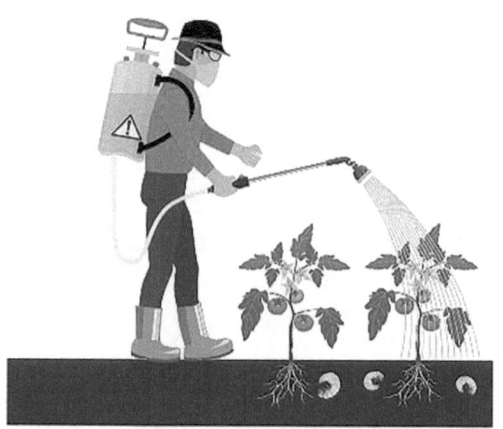

Keep your body absent of toxic substances. The biggie is artificial sugar and fried foods. Sugar in blood starts the process of insulin secretion. Insulin then stores this sugar as fatty deposits in your body. Males typically store the fat in their abdominal regions, and women in their breast, butts and thighs. It is the life force needed to breed diabetes and fuel cancer, an avoidable condition if sugar was eliminated. Artificial sugar trick our immune system into working overtime to remove this foreign molecule not found naturally anywhere on the planet but made in a laboratory, it's toxic and useless. So while our immune system is working over time trying to metabolize these pink, yellow, and blue chemical packages, other pathogens are being ignored and in creeps the condition of being immune-compromised. Fried foods use cheap oils that inflame our systems and damage our vessels. This causes a fast downward health spiral. Add crushed nerves, locked joints, daily stress with a side of laziness—a recipe for disaster.

"It is easy to dodge responsibilities, but we cannot dodge consequences of dodging responsibilities." (B. J. Palmer, DC)

Change can happen now! Nothing will have a greater impact on your future than the changes you start to implement on a daily basis today. Each time you make a choice you move toward or away from a particular goal, direction or destiny. Choices can be wiser and become the bridge you build toward the better future you desire. You are in charge of your own wellness destiny.

"Your body is your temple.
Keep it pure and clean for the soul to reside in."
(B.K.S. Iyengar)

Your body is a blank canvas; choose wisely what you put in it, on it and how you may be neglecting it. I know you will love the masterpiece you create on your very own canvas. Step by step, action by action, good decisions compounded over time yields magnificent results that are measureable not by just scales, blood pressure, etc. But by the life gained, which is worth its weight in gold, active thriving and vibrant! I am excited about what has been revealed to you so far in this book but yet there is so much more ahead, keep pressing forward, and share this great information with a loved one so they may benefit also.

"God can give you the strength to keep pressing
forward through the times of trials and pain. God
calls us to remain faithful, keep our integrity intact
and respond by trusting in Him. He will see us
through the storms of life." (Jeff Trigo, D.C.)

I highly recommend Love Me Nutrition supplement products. Live healthy, live longer. www.LoveMeNutrition.com

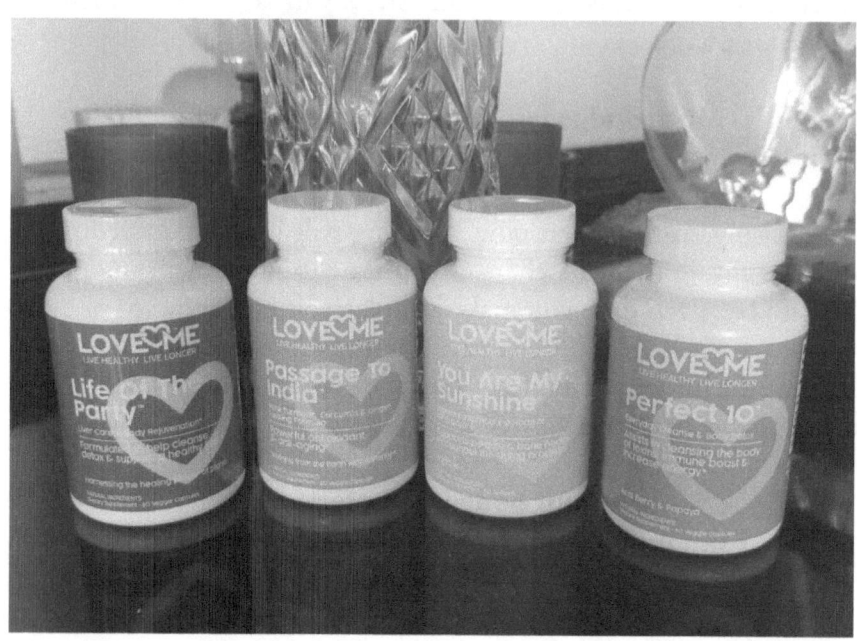

Boosting your God given natural immunity with chiropractic adjustments on a regular basis, daily whole food supplementation, regular exercise, adequate rest, the alkaline diet, anti-oxidants, probiotics and periodic fasting; will help you to avoid and or combat disease. Wellness is earned by deliberate actions taken over the course of time. Expression of life can only freely flow through a well-tuned, well-adjusted spine. Spinal neglect will yield loss of function, spinal decay, distortion, dysfunction, and disease in any individual. Remember ALL spines get locked segments called Vertebral Subluxation Complex, (VSC) and spinal neglect is a sure way to welcome loss of vitality and function. Ask yourself this question, do you have a wellness plan?

"If you're looking for inspiration, wisdom, truth and understanding, read the best self-help book ever written, The Bible." It's the living WORD of God! (Jeff Trigo, D.C.)

CHAPTER 5

Natural Remedies

There is so much to be said when talking about the many natural different methods available today that aid and assist us in the healing process. I believe the most important one, besides prayer, which should be at the top of the list, is prevention. The dental field hit a home run with getting this message across to the public in regards to cavity prevention; brush and floss your teeth daily and you will most likely not get a cavity! If you ignore your teeth then the consequences are painful and costly. Well, we can get a new tooth but not a new spine! Why are people neglecting their spine? Chiropractors failed to hit this same education homerun and therefore only adjust 10 percent of the population today! The spine allows the master system to travel through specific holes made for nerves. Locked spines close down the size of these holes and crush nerves. This subluxation controls our health's destiny via our nerve functions; it's either power on or off. Also without motion our spine rots away while getting labeled as arthritis. I have witnessed this process happening in as quickly as eleven years of neglect.

I have before and after X-rays of a woman who was seen by one of my colleagues. He recommended a treatment plan to help her with her chronic head, neck, shoulder and hand pain. She decided against the chiropractic treatment plan and wanted quick results regardless of any possible side effects. She began pain management medications, cortisone shots, and physical therapy. She ignored the cause along with her medical team, and during this course of care everybody ignored the cause, VSC! Eleven years later she returned hurting more than ever, and the new X-ray showed that three of the healthy discs on the prior film were now completely decayed, degenerative, and dehydrated. Phase 3–4 degenerative disc disease (bone on bone), with stenosis, spurs, loss of curve, arthritis, and the fusion process well underway. This should not have been! The quality of her life has been greatly reduced, now she suffers from really bad arthritis in her hands, chronic head, neck, shoulders, elbows, wrists, and finger pain and so forth; this is really upsetting and it's happening all over the world!

One of the main promoters of our great chiropractic profession said long ago:

"Long and slow is education. Not weeks, months, or years, but generations for man to speak across miles and customs to touch other men's minds enough to change them permanently into better habits of health, living and thinking." (B. J. Palmer, DC)

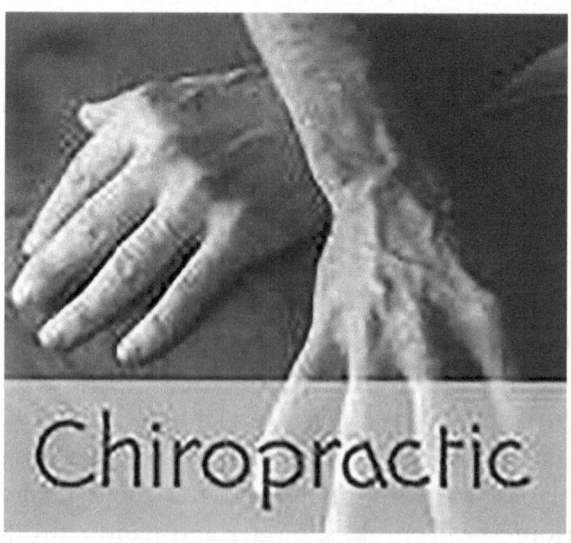

Prevention is paramount. Regular spinal adjustments that keep 100 percent joint motion and nerve supply functioning at its optimal levels is mandatory. If you also add to your regimen of spinal adjustments, regular exercise and smart healthy eating habits, you have now set the pace designed for the one-hundred-year lifestyle; that's what it takes to get to the triple digit mark. Unimpaired nerve supply with great joint motion (chiropractic), real food (nutrient rich) and exercise, all on a regular basis compounded over the decades. Only then will you have that great chance of hearing the cheers of "congratulations on your one-hundredth birthday."

Chiropractic spinal adjustments are such an important topic that I must continue educating the reader throughout this book's many pages. Until one can define subluxation and the importance of the adjustment! I say this because I ask my patients why you are here or why is a chiropractic adjustment important for you. They usually don't remember the education that was explained in detail on the first visit. In fact it takes approximately seven times for me to explain subluxation before they can properly answer the question. I've learned over the years to keep it simple because we learn differently via various methods. Some are great learners just by hearing; others need hands on for better retention yet others like to read it, see it, draw it, or do it.

I like to use props when teaching my patients. After all it's vital to maintain chiropractic spinal tune-ups so learning this concept via props is paramount to the success of long term retention needed to acquire wellness. Props would include having them hold a bowling ball to show how heavy the human head is (twelve to fifteen pounds). Demonstrate forward head carriage while holding the ball and moving it forward to a semi outstretched position; ball gets heavier as it moves away from holder's body. This concept demonstrates how one can get increased pressure and weight on the disc while also affecting loss of normal spinal curves, a.k.a. "The Arch of Life." Give analogies that convey the similarities of a disc being like a sponge which hold water and can dehydrate rip and tear. Use a dimmer switch to demonstrate what the subluxation is doing to the nerve as we lose more function and dis/ease expresses itself with that nerve impingement in place. Being an American Italian, I even give pasta analogies: Linguini being the unimpaired nerve, and the spaghetti pasta which is smaller in diameter, the result of a long term subluxation. By holding a spine and twisting it or moving it in a posterior position, this allows them to see the nerve getting pinched then immediately lowering the lights with a dimmer switch to demonstrate neuroelectrical compromise. I challenge all chiropractors to be animated, and pop your important words. Point, tell, and explain and educate! The garden hose analogy, when a car is parked on a hose the water flow is greatly diminished. Spray bottles too, when I talk about Masha and Dasha, conjoined twins who got sick separately challenging the germ theory—Google it. Just a quick side bar question, are the healthiest people on the planet the ones with the most medications and surgeries or the ones without? Ponder that a bit.

"A lie cannot live." (Martin Luther King)

Natural remedies are abundant and helpful. The following pages will offer many useful tips for various conditions in no particular order and no particular sequence, I believe the reader can benefit greatly from some of these natural remedies so read on and tell others, help me change the world one spine at a time! Education is knowledge and knowledge is wisdom, seek it more than gold.

Water, is one of the most important ingredients of the body; 60–70 percent of the body is water therefore please drink natural spring water, it contains natural minerals in it for proper human function. Half your body weight in fluid ounces needs to be consumed daily. Two hundred-pound person drinks one hundred fluid ounces of water a day, add lemon for an alkaline disease fighting edge.

These are the very important times that really benefit your health when drinking water, for example:

2 glasses of water upon waking up in the am, this helps activate internal organs; before, during and after exercise, especially if heavy sweating is involved.
1 glass 30 minutes before a meal, this aids in better digestion.

1 glass before taking a bath, this helps with blood pressure regulation.

1 glass before bed, keeps blood volume up, and lowers chances of heart attack and stroke. Drink often and frequently throughout the day and watch your fatigue fade away.

Water is the best blood thinner on the planet and coffee, alcohol, sodas, teas, caffeine products like chocolate, etc., are all diuretics, which cause water loss. How will you know if you are dehydrated or not? A helpful way is monitoring the color of your urine. Clear urine is hydrated; yellow is dehydrated unless a pill supplement is causing you to have bright yellow urine.

Another way is the Turgor Pinch Test. Pinch the back of your hand's skin together then let go. The skin should rapidly spring back to its unwrinkled state. A slow moving crumpled up skin trying to go back to normal is definitely dehydrated. Millions of times the patient will present to the doctor and they will have their blood pressure checked often to find it high, and the sad result is a lifelong regimen of little round things prescribed with no end in sight. The downward health spiral begins due to all the "side effects." Ready, on you marks, get set, And GO! Let's the pill popping scandal begin. Enough with this sickness care mentality. Maybe the person is dehydrated or stressed out a bit? Maybe the doctor made that person wait a while and now said person is a bit irritated. Or white collar high blood pressure—stressed out and/or nervous due to the lab coat doctor investigating you. I got news for you; the blood pressure should be checked three different days in a row all while in a relaxing environment, completely calm, cool and properly hydrated. Then take an average of those three different days to reveal a more accurate reading of blood pressure. We would see a drop in sales in the pill market, that's for sure!

In March 14, 2007, the university of Chicago Medicine discovered that in fifty individuals that had a misaligned C1 vertebra (atlas, at top of neck), who received an adjustment had a significant drop in blood pressure for an eight-week time span... This article was published in the *Journal of Human Hypertension March 2 issue*. That's one adjustment over 8 weeks! Imagine once-a-week adjustments or two-per-month frequency, wow, safe effective and natural results.

**"He who takes medicine and neglects to diet
wastes skill of doctors." (Chinese Proverb)**

**"He who takes medicine and neglects his spine
diminishes his life force." (Jeff Trigo, DC)**

It makes sense to talk about natural remedies as it relates to the spine. So I will start at the spine's top and work my way down to the bottom. In other words Occiput/C1 through cervical, thoracic, lumbar, sacrum, and coccyx. I will list all of its symptoms due to subluxation at that corresponding level, and then after the adjustment, other remedies that may also aid in healing. Just remember the adjustment should absolutely be the first thing you try to do because it is the most powerful healing tool we can harness. Removing a pinched nerve turns the body's healing power back on, which is paramount for proper brain to tissue cell communication. Innate can't function with interference. This interference is cause by the silent killer and it is my wish to no longer keep it silent.

Subluxation Level, Effects and Remedies

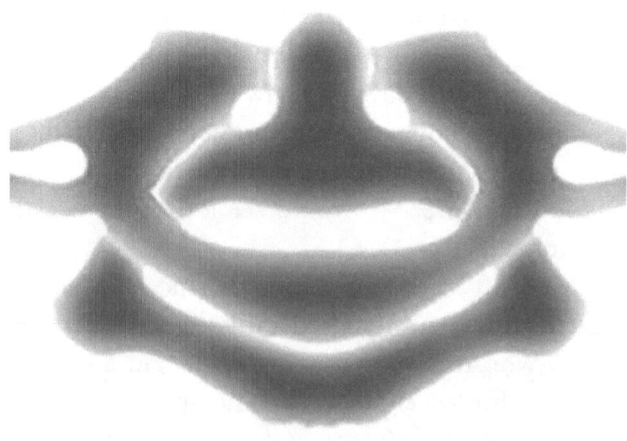

The brain stem area of the master system is the most important region that must be unimpaired to operate at optimum levels absent of distortion which leads to interference and power outage in the specialized neuroelectrical conducting function of our nervous system. As a reminder all subluxation shrink the exit site of the tunnel, space, hole, or pathway in which the nerve travels therefore causing a clamping pressure on that nerve turning off its ability to properly function.

For the doctors of chiropractic always teach the layperson with easy to understand analogies like the heart to a pump and a kidney to a filter and the spine to an electrical panel. Subluxations cause the switch to be in an off position; this makes it easy to understand. All switches may have a certain amperage, wattage or volts. You will see numbers in the common range of five to thirty. Only at the top of the panel will you find the master switches that are the ones that read one hundred and shut off all circuits. I like to explain that our spinal cord when switched to the off position, a.k.a. subluxation, causes a loss of function and a power shortage along the course of that nerve, however if you have brain stem pressure, most people do, the effects are magnified everywhere in our body due to it affecting our own master one-hundred-watt switches being in the off position. We have three switches that can cause our one-hundred-watt labeled circuit breakers on our spine to become tripped or in the locked position. These include all upper neck regions of the occiput, C1, and C2 regions. Subluxations pinch nerves, brain stem subluxation also pinch nerve but also add a choking of the spinal cord component to it. Like a necklace that is way too tight around your neck. The brain stem is similar to the bottom of the funnel at its V-neck. Imagine having a clamp on the specialized neuro tissue here. This clamp will ruin your ability to thrive. Brain stem pressure affects our Autonomic nervous system (ANS) function. It's the part of our divine design which automatically controls two important and different functions:

1. Sympathetic: flight-or-fight function (SNS)
2. Parasympathetic: resting and digestion function (PNS)

The anotomic Neuros System

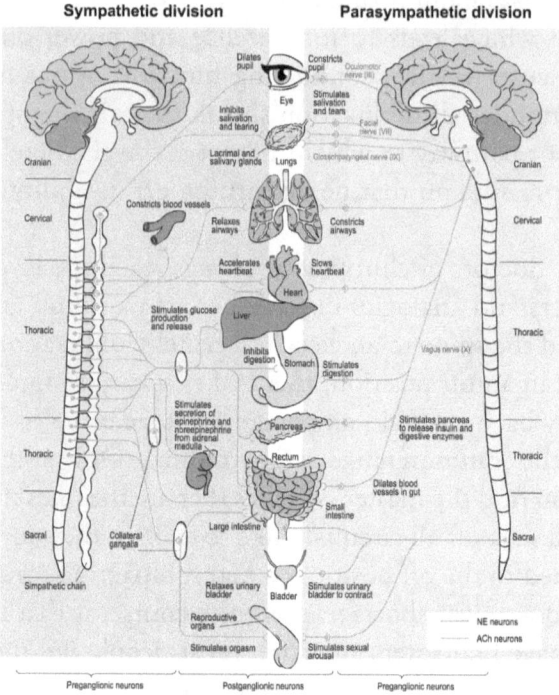

An example of this function: Imagine a nice dinner date with soft music, calm atmosphere, and pleasing conversation. Your blood is in the gut, aiding in the function of your digestive system while heart rate is normal, etc. Suddenly, crash, a door is kicked open, shots fired in the air, "This is a stick up" is yelled, you're taking cover while ducking out of harm's way, blood went to the legs and arms. Heart rate racing, adrenaline sky high, cortisol and stress levels are elevated, etc.

I want everybody to know that when there is brain stem pressure your flight or fight mechanism is excited and resting and digesting is inhibited. This is a constant condition and state of existence, stressed out to the max! One cannot live a healthy long life with constant brain stem pressure caused by upper cervical subluxation. This is simply the greatest thing you can do for yourself, find a chiropractor who will take an open mouth nasium view X-ray, and give you a gentle accurate alignment of the upper cervical region, a.k.a., the brain stem region. The skull at its base is called the Occiput or occipital bone, it's the one in the back of your head at bottom and it sits on the Atlas, C1 bone. If caught in flexion or extension it will cause so many horrible wellness robing symptoms. We are talking big money symptoms that everyday humans suffer with, therefore sending the masses seeking a cure absent of ever finding the cause; big pharma cashes in.

"One cause, one cure!" (F. H. Barge, DC)

There is a tight fit within the foramen magnum and its entrance into the central spinal column space. This specialized nervous system region of the brain stem is located at C2 and above therefore any subluxation at C2 or above, causes brain stem pressure. Spinal cord compression will excite the flight or fight mechanism of our nervous system and inhibit the resting and digesting function. As a result you will find millions in our country with various types of symptoms like: headaches, vertigo, memory compromise, difficulty sleeping, insomnia, head colds, depression, and chronic fatigue with energy loss possibly even nervous breakdowns. You are not supposed to wake up still tired and sluggish. High blood pressure and anxiety are also common with brain stem pressure as is jaw pain a.k.a. (TMJ), temporal mandibular joint pain. Sinus and allergies symptoms are also common, with C2 subluxation. Eye, and ear symptoms: lid lag, lazy eye, ear infections, tinnitus, hearing loss, etc. Brain stem pressure is also the cause of forward head carriage with extremely tight neck and shoulder muscles, if caused during birth you will see chronic ear infections, colic and possibly the development of scoliosis. Eventually expression of a weakened immunity, digestive disorders, and abnormal metabolism begins to show up. Remember we have another choice; no one is twisting your arm to go to the pharmacy. If you have chosen chiropractic and it didn't work, don't give up. If you had a bad dental experience at your dentist, wouldn't you change dentist? Now apply this same courtesy to chiropractic. If you have had a bad experience, was too rough on you, pain got worse, etc. Don't give up; there is a chiropractic healer nearby so try another. Chiropractors I challenge you to become great at the upper neck realignment. Correct all of the vectors that affect our skull, C1, and C2 regions. The ailing public needs us beyond any comprehension, who else will do this for them?

This brain stem region, which is so important for a patient to thrive, must function at its maximum level of neuro capacity for wellness to exists and manifest itself through innate wisdom. Therefore I challenge all chiropractors to become masters at it, occiput adjusting when needed, the lateral toggles, or push on C1 and the proper line of drive for the C2 which is not face down or from the head of the table, the doctor must be in that proper angle for that all-important line of drive, corrective lift adjustment needed for that C2 vertebra, or push from opposite side. I love technique; a precise, gentle, high speed, low force correction given with intent to remove subluxation. The adjustment will change many lives and change the direction of our current failed health care system that's killing Americans by the thousands daily.

So now that I finished talking about brain stem pressure and its ability to cause symptoms anywhere in the body, I will also like to start talking about the various other levels of subluxation below the brain stem, but for recap purposes I will start with the top of the spine. Keep in mind that the cause is most likely Subluxation and the effect is due to loss of proper nervous system function and joint motion loss at that level. We call it symptoms, a.k.a. loss of innate wisdom, distortion, dis/ease and lowered state of health expression.

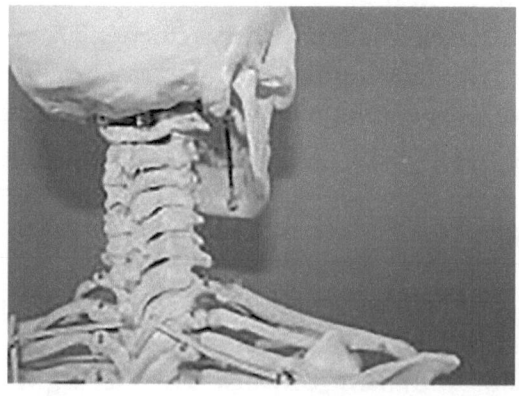

Occiput-C1 Subluxation: Nerves that control blood supply to the head, pituitary gland, scalp, bones to the face, brain, inner and middle ear, parasympathetic nervous system nerve distribution): Headaches, vertigo, pounding heart beat type of headaches upon exertion, loss of energy, insomnia, nervousness, high blood pressure, head colds, amnesia, chronic fatigue, respiratory, digestive, and immune system compromise. Forward head carriage, nervous break downs, TMJ, anxiety, top of head pain, and brain fog.

C2 Subluxation: Eyes, optic nerve, auditory nerve, sinus, mastoid bone, tongue, and forehead nerve distribution; Sinus troubles, allergies, crossed eyes, eye and vision troubles, lid lag, immune system compromise, fainting, ear ache, ear infections, deafness, TMJ issues, temporal region of pain and back of head pain.

C3 Subluxation: Cheeks, outer ear, face bone, teeth, and trifacial nerve distribution; acne, pimples especially on cheeks, neuralgia, neuritis, and eczema, neck pain.

C4 Subluxation: Nose lips mouth and Eustachian tube nerve distribution; hay fever, hearing loss and adenoids, pain by the clavicle region.

C5 Subluxation: Vocal cords, neck gland and pharynx nerve distribution; laryngitis, hoarseness, and sore throats, pain at deltoid region of upper shoulder.

C6 Subluxation: Neck muscles, shoulders and tonsils nerve distribution; stiff neck, pain in upper arm, tonsillitis, whooping cough, croup—a seal like coughing sound and shoulder/rotator cuff symptoms, dead arm syndrome.

C7 Subluxation: Thyroid gland, bursae of the shoulder, elbows and carpal tunnel nerve distribution; thyroid conditions, immune system compromise, colds, bursitis, weakness of grip strength, loss of sensation to middle finger.

C8 nerve pinching caused by C7 subluxation: 2 little fingers going numb, digit 4 and 5.

Those were the cervical vertebra and their corresponding nerve levels. Now I will begin the thoracic region, these vertebra are larger and have attachment sites for the ribs.

T1 Subluxation: arms from the elbow down including hands, wrist, fingers, esophagus, and trachea nerve distribution; asthma, cough, difficulty breathing or shortness of breath, pain in lower arms or hands.

T2 Subluxation: Heart including its valves and coverings, and coronary arteries nerve distribution; functional heart conditions and chest pains.

T3 Subluxation: Lungs, bronchial tubes, pleura, chest and breast nerve distribution; bronchitis, pleurisy, pneumonia, congestion, and influenza.

T4 Subluxation: Gall bladder and common duct nerve distribution; gall stones, jaundice, and shingles. Poor fat breakdown can also lead to dry itchy skin areas.

T5 Subluxation: Liver, solar plexus, and blood nerve distribution; immune system compromise, fevers, liver conditions, blood pressure disorders, anemia, and arthritis.

T6 Subluxation: Stomach nerve distribution; heartburn, acidosis, indigestion, reflux and dyspepsia.

T7 Subluxation: Pancreas and duodenum nerve distribution; ulcers, pancreatic conditions, and gastritis.

T8 Subluxation: Spleen nerve distribution; immune system compromise, colds, influenza, and disease.

T9 Subluxation: Adrenal and supra renal glands nerve distribution; allergies and hives.

T10 Subluxation: Kidneys nerve distribution; kidney troubles, chronic tiredness, hardening of the arteries, nephritis, and pyelitis.

T11 Subluxation: Kidneys and ureters nerve distribution; acne, pimples, eczema, and boils.

T12 Subluxation: Small intestines, and lymphatic circulation; rheumatism, gas pains, bloating, IBS, and sterility.

Note any of the thoracic spine subluxations can and will be the cause of costochondritis, a sharp shooting pain along the ribs which scares patient into thinking that they may be having a heart attack. Sharp shooting rib pain during inhalation, shortness of breath, a.k.a. SOB, is a scary symptom and painful. Adjustments will remove the source of inflammation along this nerve root distribution and remove the cause, giving the patient much needed relief.

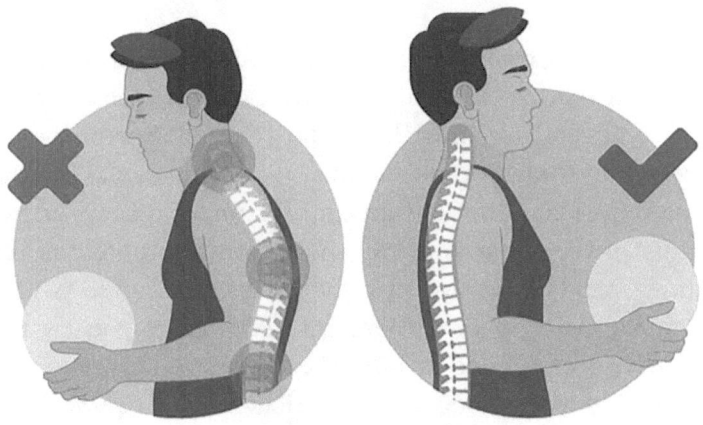

The lumbar region is comprised of five large vertebra designed for weight bearing and when subluxated wreak havoc on nerves traveling into the legs, a.k.a. sciatica.

L1 Subluxation: Large intestines, inguinal rings and groin region of nerve distribution; constipation, colitis, dysentery, diarrhea, ruptures, IBS and hernias.

L2 Subluxation: Appendix, abdomen, and upper leg nerve distribution; cramps, difficulty breathing, acidosis, varicose veins, and pain on thigh above the knee.

L3 Subluxation: Sex organs, uterus, bladder and knees nerve distribution; bladder troubles, menstrual troubles like pain or irregularity, miscarriages, bed wetting, impotency, change of life symptoms (hormones) and knee pains.

L4 Subluxation: Prostate gland, glands of female reproduction, muscles of the low back, sciatica and lower leg and calf nerve distribution; sciatica, lumbago, urination pain or too much frequency, backaches and inside calf muscle pain.

L5 Subluxation: Lower leg ankle and foot nerve distribution; poor circulation in the leg, swollen feet, weak ankles, arch of foot pain, cold feet, weakness in leg muscles, and leg cramps. Symptoms include weakness with walking on heels, a.k.a. foot drop; lateral calf pain.

The things you do today are an investment for tomorrow. The greater the price you are paying, the greater the potential rewards you can receive. If you want to know what lies ahead in your future then find the patterns in the present. The habits you form today mold your future. Are you eating as healthy as you can, not cheating but sticking to a real food nutrient rich intake? Are you neglecting your spine and allowing arthritis and disease to slowly creep in? Are you passing on your gym visits and opting for TV and couch time instead? Believe it or not, this will slowly sabotage your health and disease will be apparent. I challenge you to change today! Your spine, arteries, skin and joints will love you forever if you take care of them. Take care of your spine and your spine will take great care of you.

Sacrum: Is at the bottom of your spine. It has five holes that exits nerves for specialized nerve function of hips, buttocks, reproductive parts like testes, groin, etc. They are referred to as S1–S5 nerves. When the sacrum is subluxated walking and sitting are very difficult. Low back pain is imminent and there is the disruption of normal spinal curves which are very important shock absorbers to the spine. Weight load distribution is disrupted therefore heavy loads are now placed upon the disc material aiding in their dehydrating process. Joint motion is paramount as is proper curve maintenance through-out our life, from the womb to the tomb we must take care of our spine and it will definitely be a healthier structure for you decades later.

Coccyx: Small tail/hook like bone that hangs on the bottom of the sacrum referred to commonly as the tailbone. If subluxated, patient will experience difficulty upon sitting, and painful defecation, hem-orrhoids, itching, pruritus, piles, and pain at the very bottom of spine in gluteal fold regions.

> **"We're all on this journey called life, and as soon as we are born we are traveling inevitably toward the end of this lives journey. So the question is whether will you select a destination, set your compass and steer a course for it, or allow ourselves to be tossed around without a rudder, swept along with the tide. Please be mindful of your intention and keep your actions aligned with your goals, this will avoid letting others determine where our destination ends up." (Jeff Trigo, D.C.)**

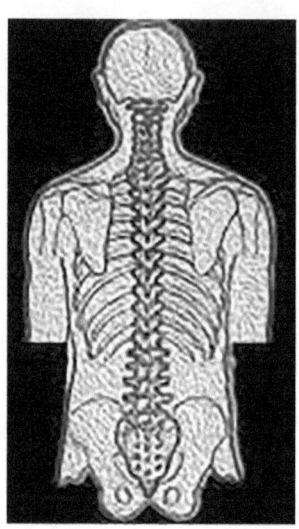

"What lies ahead in health to the sick is beyond the belief of any of us." (B. J. Palmer, DC)

After reading all of the possible conditions of dis/ease that pinched nerves can cause due to subluxation, it makes a whole lot of sense to have the most noninvasive procedure done first; the most powerful entity restored in your body, nerve supply! Get adjusted first not last! Prevention is key, you would never wait for a cavity before you started to brush your teeth well the same should be true in regards to your spine; don't wait for symptoms to get adjusted. Be proactive and take care of that 1 spine you have! Once you have been adjusted and the cause of the problem has been removed, you may want to also try some of these other home remedies and helpful antidotes that may also offer relief that are safe, natural, holistic remedies that are readily available goods found in the common home.

Aches and Pains: Chiropractic adjustments are essential for aches and pains. Alternating moist heat with ice flushes blood in and out of the region thus aiding in a shortened recovery time. Hot baths with Epsom salt ease pain. Turmeric, devil's claw, and white willow bark are anti-inflammatory. Frankincense improves circulation, and omega-3 fatty acids, found in fish oils, has shown to be effective in reducing inflammation and joint pain too. Multiple minerals will speed up healing time. Remember to stay hydrated and eat a diet that's alkaline, more on that in chapter 8. Topical herbal lotions that contain arnica, CBD, and camphor bark oil ease the aches and pains also.

Acid Reflux: Aloe Vera neutralizes stomach acids. Eat alkaline rich foods like watermelon, and drink water with lemon. Probiotic drinks heal gut. Incline the bed when sleeping. Avoid caffeine before sleep, including peppermint and spearmint they relax the gastric sphincter. Lay on left side, keeps acid away from the gastric opening. A small amount of baking soda in water will neutralize the acids. Get a T6 adjustment.

Acne: Cleansers containing at least 5 percent tea tree oil are useful with its antimicrobial properties killing white heads, pimples and skin fungus. Get C3 adjusted.

Age Spots: Castor oil rubbed on spot via cotton ball and rinsing after thirty minutes two times a day can help reduce the appearance of age spots.

Anxiety: Calm music, prayer, singing (especially gospel songs to our Creator) playing a musical instrument, reading poems, physical exercise which produces endorphins which are natural feel good hormones. Meditation will quiet the mind. A few drops of Lavender to the carrier coconut oil produce a sedative effect; rub on chest so smell rises to nose. Practice gratitude for your life's blessings. Get C1 adjusted.

Asthma: Let's revisit that new way of thinking and instead of thinking what is this asthmatic kid missing: (drug, inhaler, shot, pill, potion, lotion, crystal ball or laser beam) consider instead what deficiency may be present like nerve supply! Is there a pinched nerve at my child's upper rib cage area? They are a lot more common than you think! We all get them, SUBLUXATION. Adjust the brain stem levels and T1–3 levels. Can't wait to share my patient's testimonials with you regarding this however you will read about that in the next chapter. Eucalyptus oil drops in warm water to inhale steam. Dried figs overnight soaked in water, drink water too. Eat a combination of equal parts ginger and pomegranate, and add some honey.

Athletes Foot: Change sweaty sock ASAP. The moisture, a.k.a. sweat in your socks contains skin eating enzymes thus usually are the cause and remember to wear your shower shoes when in the public gyms and athletic clubs. Tea tree oil kills fungus and more, so mix a few drops with the carrier oil (coconut oil) and use often. A baking soda scrub, talcum powder, garlic, rubbing alcohol and peroxide with iodine are all effective. Milk of magnesia, a laxative, can also reduce foot odor via cotton swab wipe.

Bad Breath: a.k.a. halitosis. A useful cure would be to consume plenty of parsley, teeth and tongue brushing, gargling with salt water and Listerine. A Water Pik is really useful for cleaning out the food that gets stuck deep in the gum tooth crevices. Daily flossing habits will keep plaque from building up. Oil pulling is helpful; swishing coconut oil in your mouth for twenty minutes.

Bladder Infections: Increase water intake, drink unsweetened cranberry juice, increase vitamin C intake and take probiotics. Improper wiping techniques are one of the most common reasons female children get bladder infections. They need to be taught to wipe front to back not back to front. Adjust L3.

Bloating: Add ginger and peppermint to your diet to reduce gas. Consume plant-based probiotics, drink less coffee, enjoy lemon water, chew on fennel seeds or drink fennel tea, green tea or chamomile tea. Bananas and apple cider vinegar are helpful to reduce bloating. Avoid canned beans. Adjust T6, T7, T12, and L1.

Brittle Nails: Coconut oil is helpful to regain moisture. Massage it into nails. Use natural hand creams, avoid harsh nail polish removers, Biotin helps, and remember to stay hydrated.

Bug Bites: Olive oil and vinegar mixture can help take the sting out of bug bites. Oatmeal on bite, honey, baking soda, aloe vera, basil, and onion are also beneficial.

Burns: Run cool water over the burn. Aloe vera and honey are helpful. Keep area out of sun. Combine lavender oil (three to five drops) to a carrier oil such as coconut oil and rub on affected areas.

Cancer: Make sure your spine is not impairing nervous system function anywhere. Nerves are vital for immune system optimization. Must eat a ketogenic diet; because cancer loves processed foods, sugars, grains and thrives (grows), in an acidic environment. Always try to consume alkaline substances. Oxygenating the tissues like a hyperbaric oxygen chamber or wearing an oxygen mask and exercise aids in cancer fighting. Exercise increases heart rate, transporting oxygen rich blood to the tissues. Juicing fresh fruits, herbs, roots, and vegetables will boost immune system function while also eating at least one-third of your diet as raw. A diet high in anti-oxidants like pine bark, grape seed extract, resveratrol, and vitamin E, and C. Eat less proteins 50–100 grams maximum and add healthy fats instead like eggs, avocados, krill oil, coconut oils, etc. Eliminate you intake of processed vegetable oils. Adjustments to the brain stem spinal region as well as other levels in spine, vital for immune system function, are key in keeping the nerves working at 100 percent. Eating fermented foods and enzyme consumption while creating a healthy gut flora via probiotics will help your immune responsiveness and lower your body's inflammation. Turmeric has anti-cancer-fighting properties in it. Remove any toxic ingredients from your intake like artificial sugars, GMOs, herbicides, smoking, preservatives, and many other harmful cancer causing chemicals, drugs, potions, pills and shots. Undergo a detoxification of your blood and organs by partaking in various cleanses for the vital organs thus detoxifying them. Add vitamin D, because it's a common deficiency, this has shown to pro-tect against 17 different types of cancers. Get plenty of sleep and remove physical and emotional stress form the patient's life. Broccoli and curcumin have cancer fighting capabilities. Consumption of beta glucans found in yeast, oats and mushrooms. These beta glu-cans activate the body's antigen fighting cells targeting cancer cells; like natural killer cells, T cells, macrophages, etc. Budwig Protocol (a soft fresh cheese mixed with flax seed oil). Remember it's key to strengthen our immune response and fight back, not weaken it with chemotherapy and radiation.

> **"So I say to you, ask, and it will be given to you; seek, and you will find; knock, and it will be opened to you. For everyone who asks receives, and he who seeks finds, and to him who knocks it will be opened. If a son asks for bread from any father among you, will you give him a stone? Or if he asks for a fish, will he give him a serpent instead of a fish? Or if he asks for an egg, will he offer him a scorpion? If you then, being evil, know how to give good gifts to your children, how much more will your heavenly Father give the Holy Spirit to those who ask Him!" Jesus, Luke 11: 9-13**

Canker Sores: Warm salt water or baking soda gargle. A drop of milk of magnesia on the sore and slippery elm throat lozenges.

Carpal Tunnel: This is absolutely a chiropractic-related condi-tion. C7 subluxation will cause weak grip and middle finger to go numb. Make sure that there is not another brachial plexus crush site like pressure from scalene muscles, or pectoralis minor muscles. A dropped metacarpal bone can also cause the diameter of the tunnel to shrink. Rubber band exercise; wrap fingers with band and open hand to a claw like position. It's like a flower bud opening and clos-ing. This will support the extensor muscles and add a lift component thus aiding in the support in the opening of the tunnel.

Chest Congestion: Warm liquids like tea with lemon and honey. Warm saltwater steam inhalant with a few drops of tea tree oil, camphor, menthol, or eucalyptus oils in the water will help keep mucus soft and cough up able while adding an antimicrobial component. Stay hydrated, a warm water bottle on chest can ease the congestion while aiding in the healing process. Adjustments to the levels of T1-3 are vital.

Cold and Flu: Stay hydrated and drink your electrolytes. The fever is there for a reason, bacteria and viruses are temperature sensitive. The body's defense mechanism is the fever. It is a natural immune response. Get plenty of rest and make sure all the levels that affect immune system function in the spine are well adjusted. Bone broth will give you much needed fluid replenishment. Probiotics are needed to heal the gut's natural flora, especially if there is a history of overuse of antibiotics. Garlic and onions in the diet aid immune system function because they are antimicrobials. Gargle with salt water and brush teeth regularly. Air diffusers add moisture to the air and release essential oils that support immune system function. Helpful oils include: tea tree, lemon, peppermint, thyme, lavender, rosemary, clove, eucalyptus, lemon grass, cinnamon, chamomile, frankincense, and oregano. Helpful herbs to include: Echinacea, ginger root, umcka, and elderberry syrup. Rest.

Concussion: Must have brain stem region adjusted! The head impact definitely knocked out of place the upper cervical vertebra causing a choking mechanism on the spinal cord and its pressure must be removed. Future impact on a misaligned upper neck will magnify future symptoms. Ice the affected area to reduce swelling. Get plenty of rest and don't engage in video games, etc., brain needs rest too. Get back to moving sooner than later, this will shorten recovery time with symptoms of concussion. Antioxidants rich foods will help the brain and so will fish oils. Turmeric helps with reduction of inflammation and creatine can be helpful in recovery speed. Caffeine is recommended. Remember not to overdo it after impact, some rest and healing time is needed. The sooner the adjustment is given the better. Hyperbaric oxygen chambers aid in the recovery process also.

Cyst: Hot moist compress, causing cyst to fester and pop. Tea tree oil, castor oil, apple cider vinegar, turmeric, coconut oil, grapefruit seed extract, aloe vera, Epson salt, hydrogen peroxide, frankincense, garlic, potatoes, witch hazel, potatoes, and potassium iodine have all shown to be effective for treating cysts.

Dandruff: Coconut oil in hair as a leave in conditioner. Lemon juice rinse reduces dandruff. Eucalyptus oil and tea tree oil via five drops added to your bottle of shampoo. Increase Omega 3s fatty acids in your diet (fish, avocado, olive oil, krill oil, etc.) Apple cider vinegar combats yeast growth. Salt scrub, aloe vera is useful as is olive oil messaged into the hair and covered in a plastic shower cap for the night. Remember if you're wearing a black shirt don't allow snow on your shoulders, brush it off before you go out in public, remain hopeful, these remedies work.

Dementia: Eliminate all toxins, address all deficiencies, and feed the brain. Prevention is the key, stay on a regular regimen of anti-oxidant supplements (grape seed extract, resveratrol, vitamin E and C, etc.), increase O2, and eat nutrient dense foods. Add in music lessons or language learning, puzzle playing, dice games with math, and keep it fun. Get regular walking or a stationary bike, go in the pool and do calisthenics whenever is possible. Eat foods high in B12 vitamin, gingko biloba, greens and bananas for their potassium. Cinnamon, almonds and omega-3s aid in proper brain function. Oxygen hyperbaric chambers are also helpful for this condition seen in the aging public.

> **"Greater is He that is in you than he that is in the world." (1 John 4:4)**

Depression: Make a long list of the things you are grateful for and practice gratitude daily and hourly if needed. Be content with those blessings. Exercise breeds positive self-esteem and confidence. The hard cardio workout releases natural endorphins that are the feel good hormones, so get moving. Ten thousand steps a day is an active individual. Sing out loud, dance and pray to our creator and thank Him for making you. Eliminate all toxic anti-depressants and opioids that may be making you want to take your own life as a "side effect." Surround yourself with people of prayer as you detox from these harmful meds. Seek drug free professional counseling if needed. Ask your MD, what is the proper way to wean off these permanently because you want to try a safer more natural holistic approach. Pick up as many hobbies as you need until you have a winner that takes your mind off today's issues that probably won't even matter tomorrow. Volunteer to serve at a soup kitchen or homeless shelter and give back. Make sure you are getting enough sleep because sleep deprivation is a major depressant. Stop watching the news! It's all negative including the newspapers and radio news.

Guard what you expose to your mind; make sure its loving, educational and positive. Don't sweat the small stuff. Stop taking things so personally the same thing you are going through is probably happening to millions worldwide. Make small achievable goals and really big goals. Celebrate your success arriving at the destination of these goals being achieved and, remember to enjoy the journey. Brain stem check-up adjustments are mandatory. Rosemary tea lowers cortisol, increase B12 as needed. Increase your omega-3's and folic acid intake. The herb St. John's Wort has proven to help some people with depression. Eliminate sugar alcohol and caffeine while going as green eating as possible, especially raw vegetables. Go outside and get some sunlight on your skin, at least five to ten minutes a day. Strengthen your body, mind and soul to be content in where you are right now. Forgive others because this will take the weight of an elephant off your shoulders. Change can happen at any point in your life, it's up to you. Choose the mindset of living victoriously, in Christ you are forgiven from sin. Strive to give each day 100 percent effort in creating and scripting your perfect day. You are a cherished loved one of our most high God our Father in Heaven. A great inheritance awaits the believers, so remain faithful that Christ did all the work for us on that cross, bridging the gap between heaven and earth. Remember that God loves you unconditionally, always and forever. With this type of mindset, you can be sure that this will create a sense of lasting joy and happiness.

Diabetes: There are two types of diabetes, type 1 you are born with and your cells just don't have the required door (receptor sites) for sugar uptake. Type 2 is caused by a diet high in sugar for a lengthy amount of time that the body down regulates the new cells with lack of these "doors" because it is overwhelmed with high sugar saturation and therefore metabolizing it while working overtime. Insulin is therefore needed due to the cell's inability to function normally. Type 2 is totally avoidable and unnecessary, and it's most commonly caused by being overweight, obesity, poor diet and lack of exercise. The diet that is high in sugar is most susceptible. Sugar (glucose combined with sucrose) is made in a factory and not found anywhere on the planet. It has been added in so many foods and comes well-disguised for a taste benefit but brings you nothing but absolute health sabotage. Complex carbohydrates like bread, crackers, chips, fries, cakes, cookies, cereal, muffins, donuts, ice cream and other bake goods, sodas, juice, candy, etc. They are all loaded with sugar, and need to be avoided. Prevention is the key here again! Take responsibility for what you are eating.

Ear Infection: 95 percent of all ear infections in children contain sterilized fluid yet 100 percent of the time antibiotics are prescribed, why? Kids that have had many series of antibiotics need to be put on probiotics ASAP. There is a mechanical reason that the ear will develop a vacuum of pressure thus pulling fluid into the middle ear! Don't put tubes in the ear to allow fluid to drain, remove the source of the vacuum and open the drain that it already has in the Eustachian tube. C1–2 subluxation causes swelling that closes the tube on the child. When young, the vertical positioning of the tube is more horizontal and gets smashed closed just by its proximity of the brain stem subluxation and the swelling that this condition causes. This vacuum pulls sterile fluid into the middle ear chamber and causes irritation to the child. A study conducted in 1996 on forty-six child participants showed a 93 percent improvement with only one or two adjustment sessions. A warm moist compress will ease pain. Holistic ear drops are helpful; add a few drops of tea tree oil to an olive oil carrier. Ginger is also anti-microbial (soak in olive oil and add a few drops).

Hydrogen peroxide can help with external canal infections. Please get your child adjusted, kids fall 1,500 times by the age of two learning to walk and any one of these traumas including birth trauma is most likely the cause of the upper neck subluxation leading to "ear infections," which are not really infections!

Eczema and Psoriasis: Diet is an important factor as is nerve supply. Regular checkups by the chiropractor are very important. Balance gut health via probiotics. Coconut oil has healing properties. Cut out all sugar from the diet because eczema loves and needs sugar to thrive. Eat a diet rich in omega 3 and fish oils, and add flax seeds to your salads, smoothies and veggies. Tea tree shampoos, soaps and lotions will naturally subdue growth. Aloe vera will help with healing also. Vitamin E, witch hazel, sea salt baths, lavender and licorice extract can all be helpful treatment methods in these skin conditions.

Erectile Dysfunction: Also known as (ED). In order for hardness to be acquired, there must be both parasympathetic nervous system function and sympathetic nervous system function. The P "points it," the S "shoots it, or is responsible for ejaculation. There still exists a blood delivery component to the spongy tissue that fills up thus causing its growth. So it makes a lot of sense to eat a diet that is healthy for your arteries; foods that don't clog up the pipes! High fiber diets can also help clean out arteries. Eat an apple a day, and other soluble and non-soluble fibers. Lose weight and work out. Reduce stress and anxiety. Stop smoking and using any artificial sweeteners. Cut out processed foods and refined vegetable cooking oils. Medications may have ED side effects so always learn what "side effects" may be contributing to any health related issues. Limit your alcohol and caffeine intake. Saw Palmetto helps regulate natural testosterone. Korean red ginseng has libido boosting properties and acts like an aphrodisiac (sex boosting) element as does Yohimbe bark, sandalwood and rose essential oils. Niacin acts like a vasodilator (opens the arteries); and L-arginine is an amino acid that aids in blood flow. Cervical and sacrum adjustments ensure proper parasympathetic nervous system function, and adjustments to the thoracic region ensures optimal sympathetic function. Stay regular with your chiropractic appointments for best results.

Fibromyalgia: Imagine having so many falls and accidents in your life, and yet you have never been to a chiropractor. Multiple levels of subluxations exist throughout your whole spine! This will cause so many symptoms, fooling most doctors into creating a new name for this confusion called "fibromyalgia." Always tired, headaches, digestive symptoms, multiple muscle spasms a.k.a. trigger points, failure to thrive, energy loss, sleeplessness, bright lights hurt eyes, etc. These can all be caused by separate levels of pinched nerves. Studies have shown amazing results when chiropractic care was given to fibromyalgia patients and spontaneous remission was further diagnosed by MDs versus stating the real facts, chiropractic adjustments were so beneficial that they removed the cause. Remember to be patient, don't miss your adjustment appointments because healing may take some time. Trust the process, God doesn't make junk!

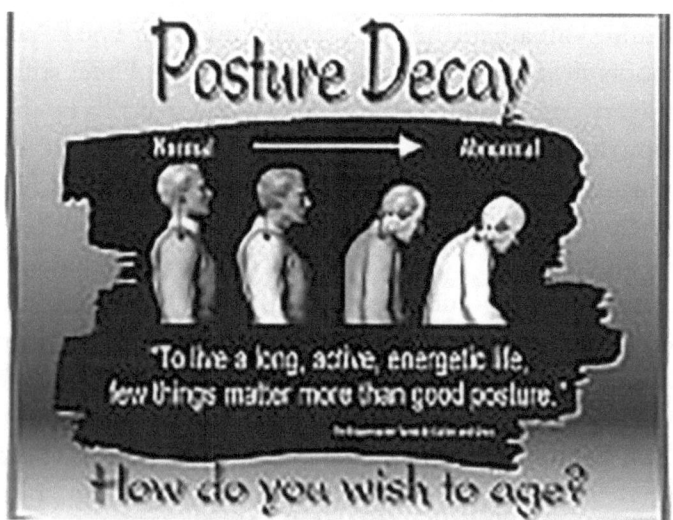

Food Poisoning: The excessive vomiting and diarrhea caused by food poisoning will deplete your body of much needed fluids and salts (electrolytes). Try to drink potassium and calcium rich fluids.

Activated charcoal will help kidney function by filtering out undigested toxins and drugs. Rest and hydrate. In regards to the condition of your food, when in doubt, throw it out!

GERD: (Gastro-esophageal reflux disease), see acid reflux but also remember not to over eat, cut out late night caffeine, chocolate and alcohol. If you are overweight, weight loss will help this condition. Also avoid raw onions. Adjust T6–T7.

Gout: Happens when the body can't metabolize purines. Purines are found in alcohol, cheese, deli meats, sardines, mackerel, liver, anchovies, scallops and game meat, etc. Eat more plant-based diets because they are low in purines. Uric acid builds up in the body and eats away bone in big toe causing pain that will wake you up at night. It will also add deposits of crystals on ear lobes. Kidney stones can be a gout complication. Reduce sugar, grains, and sodas. Treatment remedies that are helpful include black cherry juice or extract, strawberries, celery seed extract, fish oils, enzymes, and alkaline minerals like magnesium are helpful in neutralizing the purine effect in gout. Change of diet is mandatory.

Hangover: It is very important to rehydrate. Coconut water is a great hydrating fluid and contains natural sugars while replenishing electrolyte levels. Watermelon provides relief and nourishment. Eat a healthy meal. A glass of pickle juice before bed will give the body much depleted electrolytes and water with lemon adds an alkaline benefit. Get adequate rest and in severe cases intravenous (IV) drip may be needed.

Headaches: Adjustments at Occiput and the spinal level of C1 are the most effective method for treating and curing headaches. The goal here is to remove chaos a.k.a. loss of innate wisdom caused by pressure on the nerve, and introduce organized function back into the divine design. The Canadian Memorial Chiropractic College did a study on 729 subjects that suffered from headaches, 613 of them had good to excellent results following chiropractic adjustments. Posture is the window to the spine and avoid hanging your head down for long periods of time. A quiet environment is soothing and you can add moist heat on your head to increase vasodilation and blood circulation. Make sure you don't have low blood sugar or dehydration. Soft tissue work in the temporal regions, neck and shoulder muscles will reduce the tension caused by trigger points. This soft tissue work will aid in blood circulation into the cranium. Eat magnesium rich foods. Diffusing the essential oils of lavender and peppermint can be helpful.

Heart Attack/Heart Disease: Prevention is the key! Manage stress, don't smoke, eat a healthy diet and get regular exercise. Trans-fatty acids and sugars are the enemies so don't eat them. Corn oils, soybean oils are dangerous and inflammatory to the arteries so avoid them at all costs. Manage diabetes if that is applicable. Lose weight. Red wine in moderation has shown to have heart health medicinal purposes, eat a diet that is high in antioxidants. Regular antioxidant supplementation is great for prevention.

Hiccups: Try apple cider vinegar, the sharp sour taste has shown to get rid of hiccups. The diaphragm when in spasm, initiates the hiccup process, so make sure that you have 100 percent nerve supply to that region. Adjust C3, C4, and C5 the level of the phrenic nerve, which innervates that region of the body. People have also tried holding their breath, biting into a lemon, drinking a glass of water swiftly and gargling water. Boo! Did that startle you? A sudden fright can relax this nerve that controls the diaphragm.

Hot Flashes/Menopause: Black cohosh has been getting a lot of scientific attention for its possible relieving effects on hot flashes. Studies show that women who consumed two tablespoons of flaxseeds a day cut the frequency of hot flashes in half. Flaxseeds contain ligands which are estrogen-like compounds thought to help with the fluctuating hormone levels associated with menopause. A 2012 study show licorice root to be an effective treatment method if 330mg per day were consumed three times daily, and a study done in 2013, valerian root at 255mg daily three times a day for eight weeks also had favorable results. Red clover, ginseng, kava, evening primrose oil and Dong Quai are also helpful. Diets that are low in soy help reduce the effects of menopause. The average onset of menopause is age fifty-five with the absence of menses for a six-month period by definition.

Health doesn't come to us instantaneously; it's acquired and grows by great wellness choices compounded over time expressed as a thriving individual. (Jeff Trigo, DC)

Insomnia: C1 subluxation will cause many of those sleepless nights. Argh, what a drag to always be tired in the AM! After getting that atlas adjustment, make sure you limit the caffeine while staying hydrated during the day, don't over drink too late, it may cause frequent night time excessive urination urge. It is also wise to really expend as much energy as you can daily. Exercise will drain your battery, a.k.a. energy, and allow for sweeter sleep where you can fully recharge for the next day.

The sleep of a laboring man is sweet, whether he eats little or much; but the abundance of the rich will not permit him to sleep. (Ecclesiastes 5:12, NKJV)

A study in 2010 showed that people who drank cherry juice twice per day fell asleep sooner than the placebo drink. Chamomile tea, passion flower and St. John's Wort has had beneficial results with many studies. Limit your electronic over stimulation to achieve better sleep. Try mind calming prayer, song, meditation techniques, like being thankful for all your blessings in life, etc. Keep to a regular bed time routine and sleep in a cool environment. Posture while sleeping is also very important. On your back it is better to have a thin pillow with cervical arch support. On your side you will need a thicker pillow so that your head remains level. While on your side a second pillow is needed for the space between your knees to keep femur bones in proper alignment and reducing force on the hip joint. Please try not to sleep on your stomach because this causes over rotation of the cervical spine. Rotation is needed to allow for unimpaired breathing, thus causing upper neck subluxations. Alcohol is a REM robber (rapid eye movement), which is observed during deep recharging sleep, so reduce or eliminate late night drinking.

Irritable Bowel Syndrome (IBS): Gut health and nerve supply is paramount in solving this condition. The area where the ribs end and lumbar begin is the T12, L1 region. The area is also known as the thoracic-lumbar junction. The T12 vertebra has nerves that exit and go to the small intestines, L1 the large intestines. If you have clamps on those nerves, a.k.a. subluxations, then it's very common to see the pipes not working correctly. The intestines need nerve supply to do its snake like motion, peristalsis, and move its contents along its way. Without nerve supply, the pipes get impacted. Pain pills will also destroy this snake like motion and cause gut issues too. Probiotics are powerful for reestablishing gut health. Digestive enzymes will help break down undigested foods. Peppermint oil has shown to reduce pain but not provide any relief for constipation or diarrhea. Fiber may help clean out the pipes and allow for better function but too much fiber can hurt. Reduce stress, get plenty of exercise and try to eat as healthy as you can while eliminating sugars, and chewing your food very well, and drink more water. Patients respond well when nerve supply is restored by that gentle accurate adjustment.

Jaundice: Yellowing of the skin and whites of the eyes; too much bile from the gallbladder is in the blood stream. Bile is like soap, it breaks down fats to really smaller absorbable droplets. Obstruction like stones may be a cause or excessive red blood cell break down in the body can lead to yellowing of the skin as the liver is overwhelmed with metabolizing the RBCs. Treatments include but not limited to: T4 adjustment, sunlight exposure, sugarcane juice, essential oils, garlic, ginger, lemon juice, green grape juice, tomatoes, basil, goat milk, vitamin D, papaya, oregano and barley water. Eat plenty of fruits, vegetables and whole grains. Eat green leafy power foods, like kale, spinach, etc., and eat your fiber, soluble and non-soluble. Avoid fast, fatty and greasy foods.

Jock Itch: Wash the area three times a day and keep the area dry using different towels. Don't scratch the area it may cause spreading. Wear loose fitting clothes and use an anti-fungal cream because jock itch is ringworm, a.k.a. tinea cruris. Natural remedies include diet change (reduction of sugar and yeast), apple cider vinegar is antibacterial and antifungal. Baby powder to keep dry, garlic and honey is anti-bacterial and soothes itching. Tea tree and lavender oils combined to the coconut carrier oil are powerful in combating these pathogens and aloe vera for the treatment of any skin infections. Tea tree soap is a good preventative precaution.

Kidney Cyst: Over use of pain pills and long term use of non-steroidal anti-inflammatory drugs (NSAIDs), have been known to be a major cause of kidney cysts. Cranberry juice in general has a very medicinal function in overall kidney health. Regular adjustments at T10 and T11 vertebral levels, for proper nerve supply are important to maintain in any successful kidney treatment regimen. Try to eat four to five cups of fresh and as raw as possible, fruits (especially citrus) and vegetables daily. For and added edge drink herbal tea, no smoking, regular walking and exercise. Chinese Traditional Medicine (CTM), suggest dandelion root, milk thistle or corn root. Garlic, watermelon, figs, and wild hydrangea have also successfully treated kidney cysts.

Kidney Stones: Staying hydrated is the key to prevention of kidney stones. When passing a stone, up your water intake to twelve glasses per day instead of eight. Lemon juice contains citrate, which prevents stones from forming and basil juice and apple cider vinegar contains acetic acid, which helps in breaking down the stones. Celery juice removes toxins; pomegranate juice improves kidney function and is loaded with powerful antioxidants. Wheat grass juice and horse tail juice will help increase urination, decrease the inflammation and is helpful in passing the stone. Lab grade Chanca Piedra, an herbal remedy, helps break down the stones and prevents new formation of stones; it also causes ureteral relaxation so the stone can pass easier.

Laryngitis: C5 vertebral subluxation impairs vocal cord function, so maintain your regular spinal tune-ups. Rest your voice, gargle with warm salt water, and breathe this salty moist air. Stop smoking, yelling, and excessive alcohol use. Apple cider vinegar will help balance stomach acids; raw honey, garlic and ginger are beneficial too. You could add a couple drops of peppermint oil to water or tea. Marshmallow root aids with inflammation and speeds up healing, and slippery elm helps treat GERD, which may be a cause of the laryngitis due to acid irritation on the soft tissues of the throat and vocal cords.

Lice: You will need to invest into a good lice comb. Mix fifteen to twenty drops of tea tree oil into carrier oil like coconut or olive oil (two ounces), and rub the affected area and allow it to soak there for at least twelve hours, comb out lice and then shampoo with an additive of tea tree oil, then rinse. Neem, clove, ylang ylang, anise, eucalyptus, peppermint, cinnamon leaf, and lavender oil are also a useful tool yielding the same results as tea tree oil. Another recipe: three tablespoons of coconut oil mix in the above essential oils then message into hair and leave with a shower cap on for two hours. Comb out hair over sink, and while hair is still wet combine two cups of apple cider vinegar and one cup of water into a spray bottle covering the scalp and hair while using half the mixture. After massaging it into the hair, pour the rest of bottle into hair and massage hair and scalp. Rinse thoroughly and add a small amount of coconut oil to leave in hair when completed. Don't forget to wash everything in the house to avoid recontamination: sheets, clothes, bedding, couch, towels, etc.

Lipoma: The pathogenesis is still widely unknown as to what is the cause of these, however here are some useful tips to reduce and/or eliminate the size of these unwanted soft tissue fatty lumps under the surface of the skin: Hit them with a Bible is an old fashioned remedy it breaks down the fat mass into smaller ones; which in some causes reabsorption to happen, but this hurts. I would prefer one to three teaspoons of apple cider vinegar (ACV) added to a glass of water and consumed daily. The ACV helps to dissolve and eliminate the fatty deposits. Also add turmeric, sage and chickweed to the diet. Lemon juice and green tea aid in the reduction process and eat a healthy diet low in Trans-fats. Adding high amounts of flax seeds to smoothies and salads is beneficial while eliminating soy, dairy, artificial sugars, processed foods and MSG from the diet have shown positive effects for those with reoccurring lipomas.

Liver Disease: To truly understand the functional importance of the liver and all it does will leave you with almost a doctorate in pathology. So I have to limit the content here however I will definitely provide you the reader with some absolute gems. Liver disease has many causes: Hepatitis virus, long-term alcohol consumption which causes cirrhosis, and poor diet which leads to fatty liver disease. T5 adjustments help restore normal nerve supply to this vital organ. Foods and lifestyle changes to help support liver health and help manage liver disease include but not limited to: Stop alcohol consumption, eat wholesome and natural foods, and reduce protein in the diet. Increase your fruits and vegetables intake. Consume whole food, plant based, multi-vitamins and multi-minerals. An easy way to balance your diet is to buy a greens powder that you mix with water and drink. They are loaded with vitamins, herbs, enzymes and fibers. Eat foods high in potassium and limit salt intake. Consider a detoxifying liver cleanse. Get plenty of sleep. Herbs to add: Sho-saiko-to, AKA Xiao-Chai-Hu-Tang and Minor Bupleurum formula to the diet it has shown to have beneficial effects on the treatment of chronic hepatitis and liver cirrhosis. Milk thistle seed, peppermint, dandelion root, Chanca Piedra, borotutu bark, chicory root, and organic yellow dock root are all liver detoxifying aids.

By persevering through the difficult times, and overcoming mistakes and failures, you have the opportunity to adapt, adjust, learn and make the necessary changes for the better. (Jeff Trigo, DC)

Lupus: An autoimmune disorder in which the patient suffers from chronic inflammation of the joints. Please get your whole spine adjusted so that the source on inflammation is not wrongly diagnosed. Natural remedies include, chiropractic care, postural changes and corrections, diet changes, Epson salt baths, and consume these often: Turmeric, garlic, coconut oil, apple cider vinegar, basil, green tea, flax seeds, omega 3 fatty acids, alkaline diet, probiotics, vitamin D, and CoQ10. Regular chiropractic care will boost immune system function.

Macular Degeneration: A healthy diet rich in fibers to maintain circulation through the smallest blood vessels that feed the retina and other important eye functions is paramount. Include consumption of omega 3's and 9's fatty acids (fish, avocados, nuts, and olive oil, etc.) daily. And a long term regimen of antioxidant rich foods and supplements will be not only be preventative but possibly reversing this condition as long as late stages have not been reached yet. Vitamin A as well as beta carotene has always been helpful in maintaining eye health. You have heard an apple a day will keep the doctor away right, that's because apples are super foods in my opinion. Well, here is a new one for you to recite to others,

"A tomato a day will help you to see along your way." (Jeff Trigo, DC)

Tomatoes are high in lycopene which has been proven to aid not only macular degeneration, but other visual symptoms as well. Green leafy veggies are not only helpful here but need to be considered as a given for general nutritional overall wellness as is an alkaline diet and an antioxidant rich daily intake habit. Other helpful substances include but not limited to: Red wine, gingko biloba, green tea, vitamin E and C, taurine, pine bark, resveratrol, and grape seed extract, etc. It is also good to do eye exercise while avoiding strenuous lengthy time with reading, taking breaks often to focus on something at least twenty feet away for twenty seconds every twenty minutes (20-20-20 rule). This allows the tiny muscles in the eye that change the shape of the lens, to accommodate for near sight versus far sight, to relax. Closing your eyes also shuts off the lights allowing the optic nerve to rest.

Male Infertility: A healthy sperm count is considered to be 15 million per ml. or 39 million per sample/ejaculate. Healthy testosterone levels are important in maintaining healthy levels of sperm. Avoid over exposure to harmful rays like X-rays. Pilots are exposed to harmful rays while flying. Heat can cause a low count like tight underwear, frequent spa encounters, etc. Exercise benefits multiple functions, and getting plenty of sleep while eliminating stress plays an important role also. Smoking, alcohol, drugs, soy consumption and many medications have shown to contribute to a low sperm count. Antioxidants, multiple minerals, vitamin D, folate, coenzyme Q10, and zinc support and maintain healthy male function. Herbs that help include: Ginseng, turmeric and fenugreek. Foods: Walnuts, bananas, fish, garlic, broccoli, dark chocolate, red wine, dark leafy greens, fish, oysters, citrus, whole grains, and fermented nuts and seeds. L3 vertebra needs to be checked for misalignment that causes endangering pressure on the male reproductive nerve supply ASAP. Eat healthy, stay adjusted, and don't lose hope.

Mononucleosis or Mono: AKA the kissing disease. Caused by the Epstein Barr Virus that is passed via exchanging of body fluids. The symptoms may be delayed up to a couple of weeks after exposure. Symptoms include cold and flu like expressions, with chronic fatigue, fever, sore throat, swollen neck lymphatic glands, and in rare cases a swollen spleen or inflamed liver. Adjustments to vital immune system organs are essential to improve immune response. Stay hydrated. Vitamins A and C, zinc, beta glucan, olive leaf extract, L-Lysine can all boost immune system function. Echinacea with elderberry tea and coconut tea daily for a week are all helpful for recovery too. Bone broth is high in amino acids for a L-Lysine source. Onions, garlic, ginseng and bebeerine (found in plants) are all natural antimicrobial agents that kill virus. Add warm moist heat on swollen glands (wet hot wash cloth).

Multiple Sclerosis: The patient who suffers with this condition often reports a traumatic injury to the head, neck, upper back and/or spine. This trauma causes blood delivery to the blood brain barrier to become altered thus developing MS symptoms. Chiropractic studies have shown to be very effective for the recovery of MS patients after four months of care a reduction of intensity was observed and post MRI showed no new lesions. Follow up care two years later showed that the symptoms remained absent and this was with only four months of spinal realignments. Recovery included normal function of bladder control, leg power, numbness went away, normal gait returned, memory improved, range of motion increased, etc. Brain stem pressure was the primary common denominator in these cases and when the upper neck was realigned the patient started improving immediately. Other helpful tips include: better breathing techniques (four seconds inhale via nose, eight seconds exhale via mouth) this will saturate the blood with oxygen. Eight hours of sleep, balanced blood sugar levels, proper supplementation and essential fatty acids, omega 3 and 9s. Hyperbaric oxygen chambers improve oxygenation saturation to the blood stream proven effective in combating all types of disease.

Mumps: If infected with this virus (paramyxovirus) get plenty of rest. This contagious virus can spread so avoid contact with others. Essential oils can help like lemon and oregano oils. Drink plenty of electrolytes, soups like bone broth are helpful. Drink ginger tea with raw honey. Keep a clean home to stop the spread of the virus. Tea tree in home atomizer helps with sanitation as does hand washing and regular laundry cleaning. Epson salt baths for the aches and pains. Alternate an ice pack and moist heat for swollen neck glands. Antiviral herbs are helpful in combating this virus. Also garlic and onions in the diet will aid the immune system. Adjust the spine as needed to improve nerve supply thus restoring proper glandular function and immune system optimization.

"The cost of wellness care is so much cheaper and easier to manage versus the cost of disease care and its

associated life robbing effects. Spend a little now to thrive, or spend it all later to survive." (Jeff Trigo, DC)

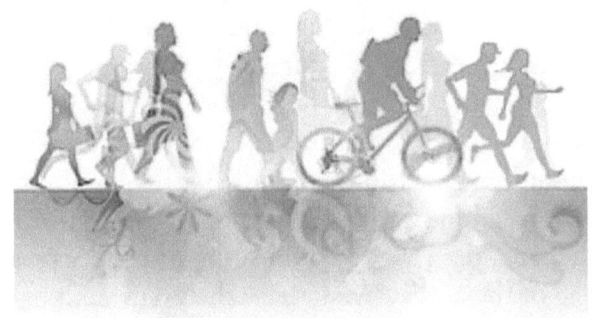

Myopia: Improving your diet has shown to be an effective way to treat this near-sighted condition. Eliminate sugar, increase anti-oxidants, and add helpful trace minerals which include: chromium, magnesium, and selenium. Boost your glutathione levels to reduce free radical build up while adding moisture to your eyes. Use the 20/20/20 rule: every twenty minutes focus on something at least twenty feet away for twenty seconds. Nature provides plenty of trees for oxygen abundance, and great view absent of bright screens, so go enjoy the great outdoors more often. Eye exercises like scanning will help reduce visual stresses. Use a holistic eye doctor when needed.

Myositis: The term means inflammation of the muscle. Adjustments to the spine will restore proper nervous system function and a great side effect is that the brain no longer sends protection signals to the muscle. Wherever a pinched nerve exists you will also find a very tight muscle that is in nervous system protection mode. Postural corrections will relieve biomechanical stresses to the muscles and tendons. Contrast therapy can also help reduce the aches associated with inflamed muscles. Multi-minerals help with cramping and twitching. Massage can aid in circulation and help with recovery time. Remove junk food from the diet because of the inflammatory reaction that it causes to our system. Rest the affected area after a strenuous workout;

creatine can shorten the recovery time. It's also important to balance gut health, so probiotics are necessary if this is a reoccurring condition. Make sure you are eating plenty of protein if this is gym related. Adjustments resolve most myositis conditions and this is seen in chiropractic clinics worldwide, so address the cause to find the cure.

Narcolepsy: Embrace your natural sleep cycles and take that power nap. Healthy supplementation habits are useful and exercise to regulate the regular recharging of the powerhouse, the brain. During sleep make sure you are on a c shaped pillow that lifts the chin up allowing a full opening of the airway. Make sure the brain stem region is clear and no upper cervical vertebra are choking off the all-important life line, the spinal cord. Join a support group to help cope, if needed.

Nasal Polyps: In most cases nasal polyps are just uncomfortable, they are not dangerous or life threatening. Eating a healthy alkaline non-inflammatory diet is helpful. Steam irrigation may be useful in treating any related symptoms. Get C2 adjusted because subluxations at that level will cause chronic reoccurring allergies and runny nose often misdiagnosed as polyps. Eat foods that boost immune system function (onions, garlic, turmeric, green leafy vegetables, and omega 3s). Stay hydrated while drinking plenty of natural spring water. Atomize some tea tree oil. Freeze a wet wash cloth in a twisted position so you can insert up nose to ease swelling caused by any possible irritants.

Night Terrors: Create a peaceful sleeping environment. Night time prayers before you go to bed, asking for forgiveness as well as giving thanks for the day and ask for protection while you are asleep with guidance and protection over your dreams. Fully drain your battery by exercising during the day so that a good recharge can happen during sleep mode. Soft nature sounds in the background if necessary. Limit caffeine exposure especially after noon. Some essential oils can be diffused into the room to aid in calming effects like: frankincense, lavender, cedar wood, etc. Hydrate with natural spring water and anoint the house with holy oil if needed. Prayer is powerful and

God answers prayer especially when two or more are gathered in His name. Remove violent TV shows from watch list.

Neuropathies: Only chiropractic can remove the cause of the pinched nerve at its origin thus providing the body's ability to naturally heal itself and return to full function. Posture corrections will support the adjustment keeping it in its normal position longer thus aid in the healing of any unwanted neuropathic syndromes. The longer the nerves are crushed the thinner they get and healing time will take longer. Regular adjustments remove VSC therefore nerves don't have enough time to express dis/ease and end stage numbness so embrace wellness care and not crisis care to avoid ever reaching this state of dis/ease expression.

Obsessive Compulsive Disorder (OCD): Chiropractic adjustments at the brain stem are a very important procedure that must happen if you want to obtain outstanding results in conjunction with the following: St. John's Wort has shown to help anxiety, depression and OCD symptoms in European studies. Milk Thistle has shown to treat this condition effectively in Iranian studies. Borage oil, a plant extract, has had successful results in reduction of anxiety disorders including OCD. Food high in zinc: fish, beans, nuts, meats and dairy aid in reduction of OCD. Exercise, healthy eating habits, music, dance, prayer and meditation ease OCD. Sunlight and outdoor activities at least two hours a day have shown beneficial in multiple studies in people with anxiety. Limit screen time, increase activity, and remain productive.

Optic Neuritis: Inflammation in one of the nerves of the eye is what this condition is. Chiropractic brain stem work removes pressure at the top of the spinal cord; this has proven a very effective treatment for sudden onset of dimmed or blurred vision, etc. Ice on the region helps to reduce swelling. The adjustment will help with the associated headache that usually accommodates this condition. Remember anti-inflammatory foods are always helpful in any "itis" which means inflammation and rest your eyes with a cool compress.

Osgood-Schlatter Disease: Kids have open growth plates still and if they do a lot of squatting, they are prone to this condition. The large leg muscles called "the quads" attach to a bump on the tibia called the tibial tuberosity. Squats put constant pressure on that little attachment site thus pulling it away from the host bone. This bump on bone gets detached. Take precautions if your kid is planning on playing catcher in baseball, doing lots of squats, or being a hockey goalie, wear a band, wrap or sleeve around the knee that supports this bone by squeezing the "bump" area where the quads attach thus reducing the incidence of detachment. Rest, ice, compression, and elevation, a.k.a. RICE, as needed. Warm moist heat will allow for an increased blood flow to the knee for better healing. Child multi minerals are suggested especially with growing athletes.

Osteopenia (low bone density): Diets high in bone forming minerals are important to prevent and treat this loss of bony density. Eat more green leafy vegetables, fish, dairy, etc. Keep levels high prior to age forty so that you have healthy mineral deposits in place before hormonal changes take place post-forties and begin to pull minerals out of the bone. Vitamin D helps in the absorption of calcium, and a little sunlight daily helps to activate D3.

A plant based multi-mineral has always been a favorite and I commonly suggest it to be taken for most of my patients. People with Osteopenia ages twenties to thirties, usually get osteoporosis as they age fifties to sixtiess. Stop smoking, increase exercise, and remember to look at the mineral robbers mentioned in the contents of this book.

Osteoporosis: This is when osteopenia get prolonged bone loss with age and therefore renamed as osteoporosis which is more loss of bone density versus osteopenia. Pathological fractures are common upon falls and flexing forward while lifting. Treatment is the same as in osteopenia. Make sure to eliminate mineral robing chemicals found in acid diets, etc. Chiropractic adjustments are always gentle and don't come into contact with the area of the vertebra that has bone loss, we contact strong structures such as mammillary, spinous, and transverse processes; all safe contact points that allow for a gentle safe corrective adjustment in patients with bone density loss.

Paresthesia: Almost all paresthesia's, loss of sensation and/or numbness, is due to a pinched nerve, mostly caused by VSC. Often they are caused by nerves accidently being cut during surgical procedures. Rare causes include incidences of lacerations, tumors, fractures, etc. With most cases, chiropractic adjustments and postural exercise can naturally restore proper balance in the body thus removing the source of nerve pressure and allowing the nerve to actually regenerate, grow and heal itself. When pressure on a nerve is removed, the thickness of a nerve can start to repair and regenerate itself over time. The amount of time varies depending on the length of time that the nerve was under endangering clamping pressure. B vitamins, CoQ10, and beetroots are useful in proper neurological function, found mostly in animal products or in supplementation. A natural organic diet and regular sunshine while getting adequate rest is also helpful in allowing the nerves the essential nutrients needed for proper function and healing. All made possible by the removal of VSC.

Pink Eye: Raw honey, breast milk, colloidal silver, and some herbal tea bags like fennel, calendula, and chamomile are helpful. Saltwater flush is also effective. Acquiring better habits of eye hygiene is important especially with those who wear contact lenses. Wash your face and eyes every morning for better hygiene. Avoid close contact with the infected person.

PMS: Diet and exercise can be useful in treating PMS. A multi-mineral will take the edge off the cramps, while adding plenty of Omega 3s and B vitamins to the diet will help to reduce PMS symptoms. Avoid bad fats, sugar and other fast foods that can trigger symptoms. Music, meditation, and stress reduction play an important role also. Mentally acknowledge the monthly timing to prepare oneself in advance so that you won't hurt your loved ones or make too much meaning out of the small stuff as hormone levels are fluctuating during these times just prior to menstruation. Love yourself and love others and pray, this will make the days easier to tolerate.

"Success consists of going from failure to failure without loss of enthusiasm." (Winston Churchill)

Pneumonia: Salt water gargle can help with mucus in throat. Get plenty of rest and hydrate with water and soups. Peppermint fenugreek and eucalyptus tea can aid in reduction of symptoms. Adjustment to the spine at the levels of T1–3 is mandatory for proper lung function. Get the brain stem region also checked for VSC. Caffeine can help open up the airways and aid in breathing. Ginger or turmeric tea for chest pains, garlic and onions to boost immune system function and breathe in the air from a diffuser with tea tree oil and Echinacea for a microbial fighting edge if needed.

Polymyalgia: The word means "many muscle pains." Chiropractic adjustments to the whole body, rest, proper hydration, multi-minerals, greens drinks, Epson salt baths, and massage ease the pain. Make sure you are eating a natural diet that supports immune system function and is not acidic which promotes inflammation. Pineapple is also a natural anti-inflammatory and should be consumed as needed. Omega 3s and 9s aid in proper body function thus reducing aches and pains. Add turmeric to foods for reduction of inflammation. After the adjustments slowly introduce light movement back into all regions of the body; like swimming, biking, walking, etc.

As you accomplish many of your small goals, you'll be moving closer to achieving your purpose and developing your potential in life. (Jeff Trigo, DC)

Psoriasis: Elimination of sugar from the diet will be effective in prevention of this skin disorder. Turmeric with its anti-oxidant properties and piperine, found in black pepper combined with curcumin aids in 2000 percent increased bioavailability inflammatory relief. For skin relief, use aloe, apple cider vinegar, and oats. Omega 3s will reduce inflammation. Get plenty of rest. Coconut oil with a few drops of tea tree oil apply to affected areas as needed. Epsom salt and dead sea salt water baths provide relief while contributing to reduction of skin rash. Tea tree soap will help with skin maintenance and prevention. Adjustments to C3, T11 have shown to be effective. Don't forget to eat the rainbow to aid in healthy skin.

PTSD: Posttraumatic stress disorder, common amongst combat veterans that recently served our country. After tour it's very important to get plugged in a support group and prayer group. Vets that you can golf with, study the Bible with, etc. Regaining trust is a very important first step. Full spine adjustment to make sure the flight or fight mechanism is turned down while assuring that the proper resting and digesting function is being optimized. Balance gut health with probiotics and eat healthy natural diets. Plenty of exercise will allow for natural endorphins to be freely produced. Prayer, music, and counseling as needed to regain trust in society and people, absent of war. Anger management classes, with peers that have recovered and have been through similar circumstances are recommended. Family and social friends that support you are very important and useful especially if they are in therapy with you. Meditation and yoga can help reduce symptoms. Avoid isolation and encourage healthy lifestyles while reducing stress. If you have suffered loss of limb or function, press on. Your Father God in Heaven loves you and be encouraged to persevere and press on because one day you will be an inspiration to others. You are absolutely loved and have a valid passport to heaven through Faith in Christ, God's only begotten Son, therefore celebrate each day.

Raynaud's syndrome: Fingers and toes go white and/or blue with cold exposure. Care includes warm water over affected areas, B3 for vasodilation of arteries, anti-oxidants to assure healthy cardiovascular integrity. Take gingko biloba to increase circulation into the toes and fingertips. Wear protective clothing, avoid caffeine and stress, exercise regularly and eat alkaline foods. Never smoke! Get adjusted and have your posture evaluated for proper biomechanics. In patients with scleroderma, this is one of the five presentations we can observe with this condition.

Restless leg syndrome: Adjustments to the lumbar spine assure proper lower extremity nerve supply. It's also good to establish regular sleeping habits, wear loose fitted clothes, take plenty of minerals so that the body is not cramping up, etc. Piriformis stretches for proper blood flow and drainage to and from the leg is helpful. Hit the iron supplements and iron at the gym because plenty of exercise does the body good. Always eat healthy and use moist heat as needed to increase blood flow and oxygen delivery to the muscles. Massage helps reduce symptoms also. Drink more natural spring water.

Reye's syndrome: Avoid giving your child aspirin or aspirin like products because they are the cause of this syndrome. Look for these names on labels and avoid them: Acetyl salicylic acid, Acetylsalicylate, Acetylsalicylate acid, Aluminum acetyl salicylate, Ammonium salicylate, Amyl salicylate, Arthropan, Benzyl salicylate, Butyloctyl salicylate, Calcium acetyl salicylate, Choline salicylate, Ethyl salicylate, Lithium salicylate, Methyl salicylate, Methylene disalicylic acid, Octisalate, Octyl salicylate, Phenyl salicylate, Procaine salicylate, Sal ethyl carbonate, Salicylsalicylic acid, Salicylamide, Salicylanilide, Salicylsalicylic acid, Santalyl salicylate, Santalyl, Sodium salicylate, Stoncylate, Strontium salicylate, Sulfosalicylic acid, Tridecyl salicylate, Trolamine salicylate. These are found in many items, so read labels. Always eat natural foods, Epson salt baths with lavender oils. Ginger turmeric and other anti-oxidants aid the body in recovery and prevention. Stay hydrated, drink bone broth, and get plenty of rest. Educate don't medicate. Remember to have your child adjusted too. They fell 1,500 times by the age of two learning to walk and run, therefore their spine is definitely locked up at multiple spinal levels robbing the child of innate wisdom.

Ringworm: Apple cider vinegar, garlic and turmeric cream are helpful in killing ringworm. Anti-fungal oils like lavender, tea tree, oregano, and calendula work wonders too. Keep areas clean of sweat and dirt to avoid future exposure. Change socks often. After work-outs, shower right away. This will prevent the sweat and dirt from harming your skin. Use tea tree soaps and shampoos.

Rosacea: An often embarrassing flushing of blood causing increased redness usually on the cheeks or nose can be treated naturally by applying lavender oil on the skin, which eases inflammation. Other helpful tips include: Licorice extract which reduce redness, feverfew plant which prevents blood pooling, green tea and other anti-oxidants like grape seed extract, vitamin C, E, and pine bark, etc. The anti-aging properties of these anti-oxidants help maintain the integrity of the blood vessels. Oatmeal acts as a protectant and exfoliates. Chamomile is anti-inflammatory and is useful in creams to help reduce redness. Keep your sheets clean by washing them weekly and read labels on face products, no chemicals. It's best to keep out of the sun or wear a natural chemical free sunblock. Avoid alcohol, stress, caffeine, fried foods, and other acidic foods including foods with added sugar.

Scoliosis: A spine should be straight when looking at it from the front or back, and from a side view it has its natural shock absorbing curves that develop during childhood crawling, etc. If the spine has a C bend to it or an S curve to it from the front or back view, this is labeled scoliosis and can be avoided with chiropractic care during childhood. Most scoliosis begins after traumatic child birth and if the brain stem and other key areas were adjusted properly at early stages of life, the scoliosis could have been avoided. As the twig is bent so grows the tree. Hint: is the child having reoccurring ear infections or has colic, cries a lot, then brain stem pressure caused by upper cervical VSC is present. Even as an adult, chiropractic can help reduce the angles of defect in the scoliosis thus creating lots of relief and stability while abating further tilt. Postural exercises to reduce the C- or S-shaped angles aid in scoliosis reduction and correction while combined with adjustments to further stabilize this condition. Most support braces will breed muscle dependency and create weak muscles. Surgical rods and other invasive procedures should be avoided like the plague. One must always seek out the most helpful, non-invasive procedures prior to invasive fusions robbing the chance of that person having a long normal healthy pain free life. When it comes to scoliosis, prevention is the key!

Sepsis: This is a life-threatening infection of bacteria present in the blood stream and prevention is best. Natural anti-inflammatory diets and anti-oxidants are helpful to boost immune system function along with chiropractic wellness visits for optimal nervous system function. Other tips include not abusing antibiotics which can breed super bugs that are resistant. Hygienic habits, proper wound care, probiotics, zinc and selenium, which boost immune system function. Propolis supplement, a.k.a., bee glue, aids in prevention and treatment of sepsis shock. Fluids are essential, an IV may be needed, drink lots of water. Prevention is best if you get sepsis, hospitalization may be necessary. Avoid pain pills, they cause constipation making the intestines susceptible to rupture with minor movements like sneezing, coughing, etc.

Shingles: This is a viral infection that lives on your skin and it's the same one that causes chicken pox. As always a healthy diet and chiropractic adjustments can be helpful especially at the T4, C3, and T11 areas. Ice and cool water oatmeal baths are helpful in reducing pain and aids in hygienic purposes. Herbal lotions, lemon balm, calamine lotion, oregano oil, coconut oil, zinc cream, green tea, and a diet high in omega fatty acids and natural vitamins including garlic and onions boost natural immunity. To reduce irritation wear loose fitted clothing; 500mg of L-lysine helps fight the virus and get plenty of Vitamin C and zinc. Also, avoid the shingles vaccination scam that spreads this virus thus creating large exposures and big sales. You don't want anything injected directly into your bloodstream bypassing the normal portals of entry and interacting directly with your vital organs. People, this is not scientific, it's sickness care, opposite of wellness care.

Sinus infection: C2 subluxation is the most common cause of sinus dysfunction and often goes ignored. Get C2 adjusted and watch that problem disappear. You must have 100 percent nerve supply functioning at optimal capacity if you want to have a normal functioning sinus. Tea tree oil and other anti-microbial oils can help clear out any possible bacteria or viruses that may be present. Hot and cold compresses ease sinus pressure. Healthy eating is always a factor for health. Breathing in a warm water steam mist will loosen up mucus with drops of a lung enhancing essential oil like eucalyptus, peppermint, tea tree and licorice. Take anti-oxidants, eat your greens and zinc can boost immunity. Adjustments are the key here, without nerve supply the sinus can't function with 100 percent communication and wisdom from the brain.

Skin tags: Tea tree oil, oregano oil, vitamin E oil or apple cider vinegar can be used by adding a few drops to a cotton ball and applying directly on the elevated skin tag and repeat for a few days maybe even a few weeks depending on size. With the oils mentioned above, use a carrier oil such as coconut oil to dilute. Iodine drops applied only on the skin tag will dry it out. Make sure you apply coconut oil around non-tag surrounding areas for a protective barrier from the iodine which is placed only on the tag itself. Crushed garlic oil and a bandage is a popular choice, some odor present, but effective none the least. Banana peel or papaya peel with a drop of tea tree oil has been shown to be effective in removing skin tags. Freezing them off is also a conventional way of removing these unwanted skin growths.

Sleep apnea: The most effective way to treat sleep apnea is to lose the extra weight that your neck can gain putting mechanical stress on the throat and windpipes. Neck sizes should be smaller than seventeen inches for a man and fifteen inches for a woman. If there is excess weight and larger neck sizes, this puts you at risk for many conditions besides sleep apnea. Exercise daily and eat healthy to lose weight. Avoid bad fats, sugar, smoking and alcohol consumption. Cervical pillows that support the neck curve can help open airways and a semi elevated sleep position is also helpful. Avoid taking sleeping drugs because they are harmful to your wellbeing. Make sure your brain stem area is clear and free from VSC.

Spinal stenosis: All subluxations cause spinal stenosis therefore only the chiropractic realignment/adjustment will restore the proper size of the inter-vertebral foramina (IVF). Failure to refer out for a chiropractic adjustment and recommending laminectomies, cortisone shots and other invasive procedures should be considered malpractice. A healthy diet will help assure proper healing but this is only after the adjustment is given to remove the cause of the pinched nerve. Note: Stenosis is the result of life's many traumatic impacts creating subluxations. VSC reduces the diameter of the I.V.F. which can be observed on X-ray. The Windsor studies, chapter 7, proves that the misaligned spine can rot away in two decades or less. Traction, postural correction, disc decompression and corrective chiropractic adjustments will be needed. Phase 3 degenerative disc disease responds well with long term chiropractic care. I have before and after X-rays that reveal the return of disc height, stenosis reduction, and increased range of motion to the vertebral segments.

Stomach flu: Adding ginger, mint, peppermint or lemon to water can help reduce inflammation and provide relief for gas and bloating. T4–7 and T12–L1 adjustments will assure proper nerve flow to the digestive regions. It is always a good idea to take probiotics not just for stomach flus but for overall gut health. Eating an unripe banana helps with absorption of extra water in GI, thus aiding in reduction and/or elimination of diarrhea. Carrots are high in Vitamin A, which helps to reduce gut inflammation and fight off the virus so supplementation of vitamin A is helpful. Replenish your electrolytes with coconut water, bone, chicken or vegetable broths. Stay hydrated, drinking plenty of natural spring water, which is always a healthy habit.

Stomach ulcers: Foods to avoid include alcohol, hot chili peppers, fried foods, milk chocolate, tomatoes and other foods high in acid. If you have normal sugar levels, honey can aid in stopping the bacteria thrive that lives amongst ulcers. Probiotics help gut functions.

Foods that will help heal your ulcers and gut include: Berries, black olives, dark chocolate, flax seeds, cranberries and their extract, garlic and other alkaline foods like kale, broccoli, apples, red grapes and legumes. T4–7 and T12–L1 adjustments will aid proper digestive neurological support, a common subluxation area that when present, GI function is greatly compromised.

Strabismus: AKA crossed eyes, it's important to have the brain stem region adjusted. Eye exercises are useful in building strength in the muscles that move the eye ball. Exercises can include tracking or looking at objects as you bring it closer to the bridge of the nose, until it becomes blurry, then out again. Track pendulum movements, in and out movements, etc. Get that weak eye or crossed eye exercising. Wear a patch over the good eye and allow for corrections to take place as the weak eye must work harder and regain strength. Don't overdo it; rest the eye if the muscle begins to strain. Consult an eye doctor for proper exercise techniques that are unique to your misalignment before any invasive surgical procedures.

Strep throat: C5–6 adjustments are so important for proper nerve supply to the throat and glands and often remain unchecked. See the story of Paul in chapter 6. Oral hygiene is important in prevention. Brush teeth in the a.m. and p.m. Gargle with antiseptic rinses and salt water. Don't forget to floss because germs and plaque can build up in between the teeth and hide in gum lines. Use a water pik for deep cleaning and flushing out gum junk that can lead to larger problems like strep throat. Other ways to help with the problem include: Honey, chamomile tea, fenugreek, peppermint, slipper elm, baking soda, marshmallow root, apple cider vinegar, cayenne pepper, and garlic.

Stroke: Prevention is best. Natural diets high in anti-oxidants like resveratrol, grape seed and pine bark extract are all great for cardio-vascular support. Avoid junk foods that clog arteries and become dislodged (emboli) closing down smaller blood vessels in brain leading to stroke conditions. High fiber in the diet helps keep arteries clean like apples and carrots don't forget the dark leafy greens too. Cook with oils that have a high smoking point, grape seed oil or avocado oil. Get plenty of exercise to ensure a healthy fitness level and it keeps the extra weight off. Garlic, gingko biloba and turmeric in the diet help prevent blood clotting. Diets high in fish have less stroke occurrences due to the healing properties of the omega 3's. Avoid smoking cigarettes at all costs. Stress management is paramount. Ginseng helps in the recovery process post stroke. Raw juices and vegetables are great for prevention and recovery too. Some studies have shown Chinese motherwort aids in recovery by reducing the area affected in stroke patients.

Stye: Prevention includes face washing daily and before bedtime with a tea tree like soap. Treatment: warm water towel or compress will actually allow it to fester and pop. Soak a clean towel in warm to hot water and apply for 15 minutes. Coriander seeds have anti-bacterial properties and can help clean and disinfect area. If needed for pain relief, you can use a cool slice of cucumber or potato.

Subluxation: Only a doctor of chiropractic has been trained to effectively and safely locate and remove subluxation, which is a locked spinal segment. This is the most common missed, undiagnosed or unchecked source of so many other health conditions that plague people everywhere today. A series of spinal adjustments, that are precise and gentle, while low in force, given by a chiropractor will help correct this common condition. Each adjustment reduces the damaging effects that subluxations wreak upon our bodies. Each adjustment propels you further towards wellness and they have an accumulative effect. The adjustment will restore proper motion to the joint thus enabling proper fluid flow needed for joint longevity and the reversal of arthritic conditions. By removing the source of the pinched nerve; this allows your body to heal naturally from the inside out by

"We all get subluxations, don't be in subluxation denial, spinal neglect always leads to symptoms." Jeff Trigo, D.C.

improving neurological function in all parts of the body: organs, tissues, cells, glands, muscles and skin everywhere.

"You have to find the pinched nerve. You have to find the vertebra causing it. You have to have a scientific application to reposition the vertebra to take the pressure off of the nerve." (Dr. Clarence S. Gonstead) 1964 he built a 19,000 square foot facility in Mt. Horeb, Wisconsin that treated 600 patients a day. Clinic included a restaurant, hotel, landing strip for airplanes etc. A true visionary pioneer.

Sun spots: A diet high in anti-oxidants will support skin integrity and slow down the effects of aging. Exfoliating the skin helps reduce the pigmentation. Natural skin lotions free of chemicals aid in reduction of age spots. I suggest you research what is in your toxic sun block ointments and creams, many of the ingredients are toxic and dangerous to your health. Mother Nature provides us with some natural items that have the ability to reduce age spots: lemon juice, aloe vera, onion or papaya juice, apple cider vinegar, horse radish, chick peas, dandelions, red currants, tomatoes and yogurt. Apply a topical sandalwood essential oil with coconut or almond carrier oil.

Swimmers ear: They have great ear plugs available for purchase for this common problem nowadays which keep the oceans toxicities out of our ears. Hydrogen peroxide is helpful to clean out the ears and kill microbes that may be multiplying as old water ages in the external canal due to poor drainage. Olive, coconut and garlic oils are helpful carriers combined with one drop of tea tree oil. White vinegar is also useful. Hanging your head in the maximum drain tilt position that allows old water to get out after swimming can stop reoccurrences. Blow dryers can dry up canal moisture. C1–C2 adjustments ensure proper Eustachian tube drainage in the middle ear chamber.

Tapeworm: Caused usually by undercooked meat and fish, poor hygiene and eating contaminated foods. I believe that everyone would benefit from an anti-parasitic cleanse every so often and I always support a healthy alkaline, immune boosting type of diet. Eliminate sugar from the diet and increase your organic eating habits. Eat garlic and onions on a regular basis. Turmeric and pumpkin seeds will kill parasites. Coconut oil, milk and pulp have antimicrobial benefits. Cloves are always one of the main ingredients in a natural herbal parasitic cleanse formula. Add 1–2 grams of crushed cloves to warm water and drink in am for 7 days. Carrots are high in beta-carotene, a precursor to vitamin A, which supports healthy gut function. Add a handful of fresh ground neem leaves to water and drink daily for a week first thing in the am. Probiotics aid in gut health. It is always beneficial to eat wild caught not farm raised meats. Fresh frozen types of meats kill the parasites due to the freezing process.

Teething: Babies will chew on frozen wash cloths and bite frozen, BPA free, plastic rings which offer relief for inflammation related to teeth growth. They can also chew on peeled ginger root, a tooth brush, or eat an organic popsicle. You can rub some clove essential oils or vanilla extract on the gums. Organic teething biscuits are a fan favorite. Chewable organic bite toys that are stored in the freezer, etc. Oral hygiene is important and so is bath time. Also feel free to give your baby a gentle face massage.

Tendonitis: "The word literally means inflammation of a tendon." Subluxation will mimic this condition and fool most doctors into getting procedures, shots or braces that really don't work. VSC will also cause postural imbalances which apply an increased tension on the end of these muscle tendons. Fix the cause and receive great results. Chase the symptoms and you will regret it while prolonging the condition and wasting your resources. Taking time off to heal is important, sometimes repetitive motions with the existence of postural imbalances will always inflame a tendon. Moist heat and ice can be used on the tendon to shorten recovery times. Don't forget to check for the cause, which is usually subluxation causing the postural distortions and increased tension on the tendons. Eat organic and avoid inflammatory foods. Stay hydrated, soft tissue massage can speed up the recovery process also. Essential oils and herbs that help with circulation can aid in O2 delivery to the affected areas, and Omega 3s and MSM reduce inflammation. After the area is healed, ease slowly back into the exercise or work that may have contributed to the flair-up.

Tinnitus: AKA "ringing in the ears." Take precautions if you are going to be around loud noises for any prolonged periods of time by wearing ear plugs. Remove any excess wax. Avoid statin drugs which have ringing in the ears as a side effect. Gingko biloba and zinc have proven to be effective treatment methods for tinnitus reduction and cure. Plenty of water, rest and removal of stressors in your day will help too. Get C1–2 adjusted, increase multi-minerals and try pulling your ear lobe down in a sharp quick abrupt manner, this will put tension on the stapedius ligament which may be in spasm thus relaxing it where it attaches on the ova window of the ear drum abating its ringing and vibratory effects.

TMJ: The close proximity of the C1 and C2 vertebra directly impact the motion of the temporal mandibular joint a.k.a. TMJ. Get your chiropractic tune up first at the brain stem region because many of my patients that suffer TMJ pain got relief after an upper cervical adjustment was given. Avoid going long periods of time without a dental check-ups because a painful tooth causes you to chew on only one side thus creating muscle imbalances. Sleeping face down with the weight of your head on you jaw all night will definitely aggravate it, so create better sleeping postures and habits. If all else fails, have your dentist fit you for a night guard to avoid bruxism, teeth grinding, and unwanted pressure with poor sleeping positions. The TMJ can also be adjusted via chiropractic treatment methods. Ice or moist heat as needed for inflammation control. Massage the muscles of mastication, the chewing muscles, to provide muscle tension relief.

Ulcers: Stop taking NSAIDs and aspirin for a safe and natural prevention. Avoid triggers like stress, smoking, chocolate, alcohol, caffeine, peppermint, tomato products, chili peppers, fatty foods and desserts. Probiotics will aid in balancing gut health and kill unwanted ulcer causing bacteria. Maintain a healthy weight and don't forget to exercise while staying hydrated. Increased O2 during exercise elevates the body's PH levels to a more alkaline environment. Vitamin E has anti-ulcer benefits. A small amount (1/4 teaspoon) of baking soda with 5 oz. of water will combat the acids naturally. Apple cider vinegar will also help. Aloe vera and cranberry juice are known to provide relief from the pain caused by ulcers. Eat more bananas, honey, turmeric, cabbage, cayenne pepper, green tea and licorice tea, ginger, dark leafy greens, organic nutrient dense foods which are all high in alkaline PH, thus preventing unwanted excessive acid.

Varicose Veins: A diet rich in anti-oxidants (grape seed extract, pine bark, resveratrol) will aid in arterial health and help prevent the capillaries from breaking down into varicose veins. Maintaining healthy muscle tone to your legs can not only be healthy for you but prevent these unwanted spider web looking veins from showing up on your skin.

Foods that support circulation are also helpful like: Apples, citrus fruits, garlic, parsley, cayenne pepper, include high fiber foods, also food containing flavonoids, and foods high in potassium. Skin massage with olive oil and a few added drops of vitamin E for reduction of appearance. You can also include witch hazel and butchers broom for topical treatment.

Vertigo: The atlas (C1) adjustment is the most effective treatment method for finding and removal of the cause. It's very common to have this condition misdiagnosed and be labeled as "the crystals in your ear" being out of position. Swelling at the brain stem will absolutely lead to vertigo caused by subluxation, therefore get adjusted ASAP for safe and fast long lasting results. Stay hydrated while maintaining healthy blood sugar levels via fruits and vegetables.

Vitiligo: Decreasing oxidative stress has shown to stop the spread of this depigmentation of the skin, grape seed extract, pine bark, and gingko biloba are a few great anti-inflammatory remedies for this. Also basil leaves mixed with lime juice aid in the production of the chemicals that form pigmentation on the skin, apply daily for a couple of seasons. Anything that helps with melanin production on the skin will aid in re-pigmentation of the light skin areas, like psoralen seeds and tamarind seeds mixed and applied topically on the skin, this mimics melanin production and aids in darkening the regions affected. A diet rich in zinc, vitamin B12, C, D, folic acids, aloe vera, and beta carotene will aid in immune support giving your body the best ability to fight against this depigmentation of the skin. Adjustments to the whole spine ensure proper nerve flow and overall improved function everywhere throughout the body thus enhancing the quality of life in general.

Warts: Mince some garlic and clove together and apply the paste to the wart two times a day, this process may take a few weeks because warts have deep roots. The inside of a banana peel is effective when rubbed on the Human Papilloma Virus (HPV) nightly for a few weeks. Freezing them off with liquid nitrogen is a common fast and effective way to kill the wart. Honey on the wart covered in a band aid over night for a few weeks also is helpful. Apple cider vinegar and tea tree oil helps stop the growth while aiding in the warts demise.

Whooping Cough: Chronic coughs have gone away with adjustments to the brain stem region, C6, and lung regions T1–3. After getting checked for VSC, try these helpful natural remedies: Turmeric is said to be one of the most powerful herbs in combating and reversing disease so always use this in your kitchen for adding flavor to your foods. Eat lots of garlic, onions and ginseng too, they aid in antimicrobial function while boosting immune system optimization. Taking raw honey will also sooth the throat while reducing mucus secretion. Tea tree oil in a diffuser will aid in lung health, add a few drops of oregano oil, peppermint oil and cedar wood oil as well. Always stay hydrated and get plenty of bone or chicken broth. A healthy regimen of probiotics will always be a good ideal especially if you have taken antibiotics in the recent past. This will boost natural gut flora for better immune and digestion system function. Rest as needed, this will allow the lungs to get healthy again.

Xerosis: A.k.a. dry skin, the best way to treat this condition is using coconut oil. These dry red scaly patches are usually due to over exfoliating (scrubbing) your skin, use of excessively hot water, exposure to harmful chemicals, dehydration and dry air. Use moisturizers that are natural and have plant based oils in them, olive, coconut, almond, avocado oil, etc. Oatmeal baths have helped this skin condition. Also make sure you are eating plenty of healthy fats like omega 3s and 9s. It's also a good practice to wear gloves when washing dishes or working with chemicals to avoid dry scaly skin. Always eat a diet high in anti-oxidants because this helps slow aging and beautifies skin from the inside out.

Yeast Infection: If a doctor gives you antibiotics and you believe that your body is too weak to combat any "infection" disease that it may be expressing thus accepting the prescription and filling it, then get probiotics too because all antibiotics will always lead to a yeast infection for females if probiotics are ignored. Also helpful is coconut, tea tree and oregano oil, boric acid, apple cider vinegar, Yakult drinks, yogurts, and hydrogen peroxide. I had a hand surgery and was given a script for antibiotics, I never filled it; instead I kept the wound clean and continued the lifelong pursuit of eating a healthy diet. I was completely fine without the antibiotics. I also didn't fill any of the pain medication scripts either. Pain medication seems to always be over prescribed!

Zits: During adolescence, hormonal changes are seen as well as an increase in facial oil and sweat production. Face washing becomes a two-per-day minimum requirement. A good bar of tea tree soap will do, don't use a soap that leaves a film behind. Face washing will keep the pores clean and prevent facial zits. Get chiropractic adjustments at the levels of C3, T4, and T11. Spot treating with tea tree oil is useful and eating real pure foods will prevent excessive grease consumption found in fast food. Get plenty of antioxidants and greens in the diet, stay hydrated and let your skin have some minor exposure time to sunlight. It's ok to pop the white and black heads; this has to happen to remove clogged pores, they release easier after a warm wet wash cloth has been applied and soothing the area beforehand. Exfoliate the area; this will remove unwanted germs and old skin cells bringing about a clearer result.

"A merry heart does good, like medicine, But a broken spirit dries the bones." (Proverbs 17:22)

I love what this planet has to offer in regards to seeking remedies made by Mother Nature. Have you ever noticed the abundance all around us? A marvelous selection surrounds most of us with a variety of choice fresh fruits, plants, greens and vegetables being ready and available for our consumption. Stay away from the fast food drive thru. Regular consumption of fast food will accelerate you to the grave. Embrace healthy habits and just because it's free and a friend may be offering it at the local BBQ or picnic, show restraint and maintain your compound effect wellness edge by passing on the cookies, chips and cake while opting for the fresh fruits and vegetables instead.

"Along the bank of the river, on the side and that, will grow all kinds of trees used for food; their leaves will not fail. They will bear fruit every month, because their water flows from the sanctuary. Their fruit will be for food, and their leaves for medicine." (Ezekiel 47:12)

Cannabinoids, a.k.a. CBD, is a chemical compound, oil extract, found in the hemp/marijuana plant. Not to be confused with the TCH component which is responsible for the "High" feeling; the CBD component as shown in a 2013 British Journal of Clinical Pharmacology, concluded that their studies found to show a favorable outcome regarding the medical properties that follow:

Antiemetic: reduces nausea and vomiting
Anticonvulsant: suppresses seizure activity
Antipsychotic: fights against mental disorders
Anti-depressant: combats against depression and anxiety disorders

Anti-tumor: combats tumors
Anti-cancer: combats cancer cells
Antioxidant: combats free-radical damage
Anti-inflammatory: reduces inflammation
Analgesic: combats chronic pain

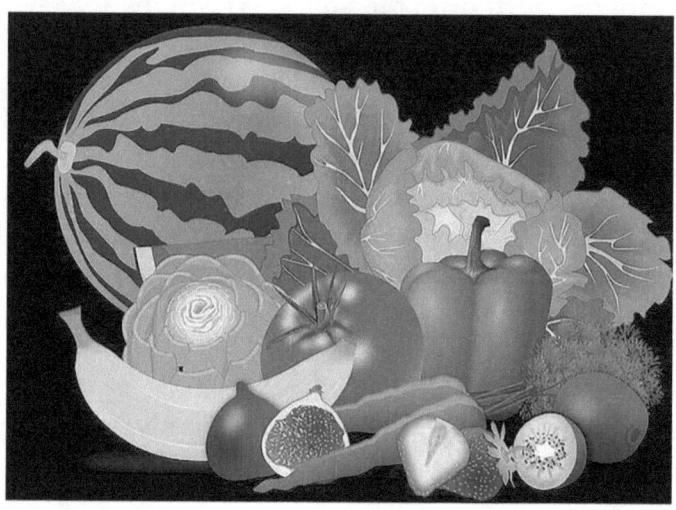

Eat real food, no boxes, bags or cans. Stay out of the frozen
food section! Real ingredients, real sources of fiber, vitamins,
minerals and enzymes are found naturally in real food.

**Enter into His gates with thanksgiving, And into His courts
with praise. Be thankful to Him, and bless His name. For
the Lord is good; His mercy is everlasting, And His truth
endures to all generations. (Psalms 100:4–5 NKJV)**

**We go astray when we attempt to do spiritual
work without spiritual power. (A.W. Tozer)**

CHAPTER 6

Powerful Pisiform

O h, what a magnificent and powerful tool we Chiropractors have the blessed privilege to use, the pisiform. It is one of our eight carpal bones located in our hand or wrist, which collectively make up the carpel tunnel. This pisiform, one of many contact points used by the doctor of chiropractic, is used to adjust the locked, fixated, dislocated andor subluxated joints everywhere. With the proper training, speed, force, line of drive and intent, the doctor delivers a life changing adjustment that alters the life flowing innate wisdom of the receiving participant, turning on the natural power within to heal without prejudice or discrimination to color, race, age, or creed. All are created equal and have great inner potential.

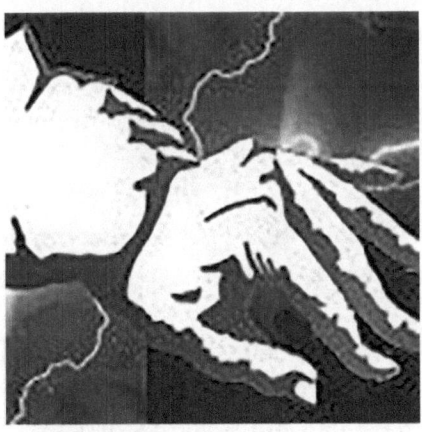

The adjustment or cavitation can make a sound when the locked joint is corrected. This click or popping sound can sound like pressure being release in a hydraulic break line like the ones some trucks have or the sound that some elevators have, etc. It is likened to pockets of air surrounded by fluid in the joints and then they sound off when released. When you pull on your finger and you hear a pop sound, well this is what I am talking about. Principled chiropractors like to reference this adjustment sound or cavitation as the "TIC." It comes from the last three letters in the word chiropract-TIC. The word TOR, in chiropracTOR, is a reference to the doctor giving the adjustment. I like to say put the "Tic back into the Tor." In other words, chiropractors specialize in the removal of vertebral subluxation complex, a.k.a. VSC. This is the only way to remove the clamp on the nerve restoring innate wisdom at its maximum potential while returning normal joint motion stopping the arthritic and degenerative process in its tracks. If you are a chiropracTOR, I plead; please make sure that an adjustment ("TIC" sound) is being given. If you are a patient, please expect a corrective adjustment that is non-force, specific and accurate, without twisting, while gentle at all times. When we correct subluxations we get to witness time and time again many miracles. Please know this; we all get subluxations so don't be fooled by its many symptoms! Fact, everyone heals themselves at their own pace, so please be patient. We adjust, you do the healing. Innate wisdom no longer has its road block; obstacles that were hindering health have been removed, toxicities and deficiencies addressed, with that wonderful TOR applying that healing TIC to your locked circuit breaker segments, you will find that this was the missing link for you to live out your maximum wellness potential, without distortion or dis/ease.

Rachael's Story: When I first met Rachael, a fifth-grade school teacher in her twenties who presented in my office for low back pain, I made her cry. I was just starting the health history questioning when she stated to cry after being asked are you married and do you have any kids? She began to explain that she has been trying to have children but they have had multiple miscarriages, and that her doctors told her that if she wants to have children she would have to go to a fertility specialist! I looked her straight in the eyes and said that's not true, you probably have the nerve traveling to the female reproductive system pinched and it's causing those miscarriages to happen. No one had ever given her hope before this day. Upon further examination I noticed how tender the bottom 3 lumbar vertebra where to the touch, typical of a subluxation. X-rays showed that L3, L4, and L5 vertebra were misaligned off the midline with wedging; In other words, they were absolutely subluxated. After the first adjustment, approximately three days went by and she returned to get rechecked.

On her second visit before the adjustment she asked me a question, "Dr. Trigo, I've been to multiple dermatologist, tried creams, lotions and pills nothing has worked, do you think your adjustment had anything to do with a 4 year rash suddenly going away that traveled across my thigh? (L3 Dermatome). I said absolutely and showed her the dermatome chart-poster on my wall asking her if the rash pattern look like this, pointing to L3 dermatome, she said yes. I was really impressed; chiropractic never ceases to amaze me! 1 month later she did not get her period and after some time it was confirmed, she was pregnant! She continued getting checked for reoccurring subluxations the whole nine months and she carried full term and had a healthy boy in that delivery room. Two years later she got pregnant again and continued chiropractic care for another three trimesters and her second healthy boy was born. Praise the Lord for this awesome gift of healing and our bodies amazing design. He used me as a conduit for her healing and because of chiropractic there is added life in this world. Remember she only came in because of back pain and had no idea that chiropractic and its healing powers could gift her life; and all of her other health related symptoms were actually caused by a pinched nerve somewhere in her spine.

The "Silent Killer" goes mostly unchecked in the everyday doctor visits as millions of people spend billions of dollars chasing symptoms and ignoring cause as they try pills, potions, lotions, procedures, bolts, screws, gimmicks, crystals balls and laser beams. Stop this madness! I suggest to you that you should try chiropractic first and not as a last resort! Bring spinal maintenance awareness to the front of the thought process, shift your thinking; we are perfect in design, lacking nothing! Remove nerve interference and get out of the way of healing.

Rebecca's Story: "Becca" presented to my office with her mother. She was seventeen at the time they decided to give chiropractic a try and they really liked my online reviews so they made an appointment. I was shocked at how many symptoms and conditions she had written down in her health history forms. This young lady has been diagnosed with almost everything from A–Z! Her mother is a nurse and had told me that it was time for a second opinion outside of the medical circus. MDs had told her that her daughter has: migraine headaches with light aura, fibromyalgia, endometriosis, irritable bowel syndrome, hormonal imbalances, TMJ, sciatica, carpel tunnel, scoliosis, and the labels keep flying off the shelves. Each Dx came with new pills, potions or procedures that will generate thousands in sickness care revenue from the insurance company. Her suffering continued with no end in sight. This poor girl literally had to massage her own abdomen approximately for two hours just to go to the bathroom. She really was expressing a complete failure to thrive. Becca was prescribed multiple medications that were literally handicapping her, rendering her hopeless, as she was lethargic, in chronic daily agony, incapable of functioning while completely feeling unstable emotionally and physically. Those same doctors wanted to do exploratory surgery and have an inside look at the reproductive organs and see if they can locate a cause of her endometriosis. That is when the mother came to her senses and said enough is enough, I want to try chiropractic. It really was a pleasure to work with "Becca," she never lost hope and believed that the body can heal itself and really understood subluxation and its detrimental effects it can have as it wreaks havoc upon her nervous system performance or lack thereof. During care I noticed that this young lady had not started to develop any breast yet, never went through puberty and when asked, it was revealed that she also had not gotten her period yet, ever. After a thorough examination was conducted to document all areas of her spine that were tender to the touch, range of motions were measured and very limited, and various other orthopedic tests were done, I decided to take some X-rays.

Radiographic evidence showed vertebral malposition at the brain stem level, lower neck, upper and mid back as well as lumbar spine and sacrum. I started adjusting her upper neck subluxations first and work my way all the way to the bottom of the spine. We got multiple bones to move on that first day. After her first visit she said the headaches intensity was way down and she was able to perform a bowel movement without any of the usual complications that plagued her for years. Care continued at three days a week for the first four weeks then a reexam was performed. Balance returned, and range of motion improved in all directions in her cervical and lumbar regions. In the first two months of care, all her symptoms were disappearing fast. As function returned, she started to blossom. Steadily, she withdrew and detoxed from all her medications, this was a six-month process. Today, at the age of nineteen, she is drug free and maintains a once a week chiropractic tune up frequency and her life has changed. Her menses are regular, full breast development and she is full of life and vigor. She is currently living in complete remission from all past dis/ease labels. Her symptom free life is now expressing wellness while thriving at its maximum potential. Shortly after care began Carol, her mother the nurse, became a patient.

Carol witnessed her daughter quick return of wellness, saw how gentle and effective chiropractic can be; and wanted the same for herself. FYI, Becca is now even enjoying employment and they are recommending chiropractic care to other family members.

Kitten: I was a new graduate living across the street from a colleague that I worked with in these fun apartments that reminded me of Melrose Place when Amy and Eric knocked on my door. Apparently one of our neighbor's kids accidently dropped a kitten and it dislodged its upper cervical spine. This poor little furry cutie couldn't walk anymore; it would wobble and fall over like as if it was super dizzy and weak. It stopped eating and playing with the other kittens and was not getting any better and after two days the kitten got progressively worse. They asked me if I could help their kitten and I said sure. After seeing which way the head was rotated and flexed, I made the call to my Chiro buddy Dr. John, and said, hi John, you ready to save a kitten's life? He immediately replied sure! I said come over and shortly later he arrived. He asked, what do you suggest? I explained to him the biomechanics that must be involved with this kitten's predicament, and the treatment needed to correct it, he said I concur, so we began. He did some much needed decompression/traction while untwisting the cat's rotation, while I applied a one finger poking impulses with the tip of my index finger at C1 and C2. I really didn't feel or hear a pop or cavitation sound. The cat and its humans left, lol if you're a cat owner you will understand that. It took me 1.5 days to pass before I was able to visit my neighbors; I was worried about this little kitten so I knocked with great anticipation. "Hi, guys," as they open the door. I asked, "How is the kitten doing?"

Eric said, "Look" and pointed to a bunch of kittens pouncing and scraping with each other, I said cool, but where is the one that I adjusted? He said it's that one there and pointed to one of the energetic scrappers. I thought I would find one isolated, being nursed back to life slowly, but that kitten had other plans, like attacking the sibling and wrestling all day. Wow I was floored how fast that little one healed and I was filled with joy, that's the awesome power of the chiropractic adjustment once again.

Paul's Story: I have plenty of patients that no matter how much I explain vertebral subluxation and the endangering clamp it puts upon our nervous system, shutting off function and starting the dis/ease process, it literally goes through one ear and out the other. Paul is a great example of this. A 62 year old friend for 30 years, knows all about my profession except when I talk I think he is day dreaming about lunch, ladies, or retirement. Nothing registers. Having said, let's talk about Paul. A month or two had passed by since I talked to my friend, so I gave him a call, hey Paul how are you doing? His reply, I have this terrible sore throat, it has been bothering me for 2 weeks, so I went to the doctor and they gave me antibiotics. I've been on the antibiotics for 4 weeks now and my throat still hurts. I told him that a pinched nerve at the C5 area in his lower neck was probably the cause; I haven't adjusted you in 9 months, where have you been? He came in the next day. Sure enough, C5–C6 was locked and very painful to the gentle touch. I adjusted that bone back into its normal position, freeing up his nerve supply so it can start working at 100 percent again, allowing him to function without interference. Within twenty-four hours his throat was 95 percent resolved and by the next day in the a.m., thirty-six hours later, it was 100 percent resolved. This was after medication did nothing for the cause of his condition. He was so shocked and amazed but being true to his nature, he drops out of care until a recent bout of sciatica showed up and now he is under care again. This is a classic example of what I call "crisis care" versus "wellness care."

Be proactive people and stay regular with spinal "tune ups" by visiting your chiropractor for wellness, absent of symptoms. Regular preventive care is the best recommendation for longevity.

Zachary's Story: I have a neighbor that used to live across the street from me and because of a chiropractic adjustment, she no longer suffers from sinus infections, and her children no longer suffer from ear infections. They stay regular with their care still to this day 10 years later. Well this sweet lady named Tina has a friend from her church, and her son was suffering from really bad asthma symptoms. Tina told her chiropractic success story to her friend Misty, who then asked Tina to inquire if chiropractic could help her 9 year old son who suffer from really bad asthma. I replied that nerves control the lungs, and that I would be thrilled to check him.

Zachary had multiple subluxations that were most likely caused by birth trauma. Birth is very traumatic both for the baby and the mother. This subluxation had to be contributing to his loss of lung function and/or asthma symptoms that he was plagued with since birth. I began adjusting Zach and guess what? Yup, he is asthma free today. What surprised me the most with this case was the big gift he brought me after six months of care! I opened the box and to my surprise, I saw his nebulizer, steroids, inhalers and other gizmos. I said what is this? The family replied that their son no longer needed any of these asthma drugs or breathing machines and that I healed their son Zach! My reply was—Your son healed himself! I just removed the nerve interference and he did all the healing. It's like taking a car off a hose I explained. I can't make the plant grow, it does that all on its own, however I can make sure the plant has all the water it needs. They were very thankful and Zach now plays basketball like his father and drums like his chiropractor.

Foster Care Woman: This case was from a long time ago approx. Eighteen years ago, so I don't remember the patient's or the baby's name but I never forget a miracle. A woman was receiving chiropractic care for a neuro-muscular-skeletal related problem, and with her was a baby that she placed on a blanket on the carpet. As I was adjusting this woman I noticed that the baby had a leg kicking type of violent uncontrollable twitch like movement. It was rhythmic in motion and it seemed like every 2 seconds the leg would bend at the knee a bit then kick and fall back down just to start all over again. This baby was approximately four to six months old. I asked the lady what's with the child's leg. Her reply was that the child was crying and the father violently shook the kid to stop and was arrested for child endangerment, taken into custody, the mother was a drug addict in rehab and that the state gave temporary custody of this child to the foster care system in which she was the guardian at this time. I said can I adjust the child to see if we can help her? She said that we needed parental permission, so no, not right now. After her third visit she was experiencing amazing relief, she changed her mind and said Dr. Trigo would you please check this little girl? I said absolutely. After feeling a bone sticking out of its normal position causing brainstem pressure existing in the upper region of her neck, I gently removed the dislodged vertebra and immediately the leg stopped twitching. The woman said, "wow did you see that?" my reply was "I sure did!"

Over the course on the next 3 weeks the baby's physical therapist said wow whatever the chiropractor did really made a huge difference because this child is now thriving again and making so much progress; progress that we were unable to obtain.

Wilma's Story: Eighty-four year old woman presents with chronic back pain for duration of two months. Her health history revealed a recent fall. She had a CAT scan and abdominal exam performed by the hospital with nothing out of the ordinary being found on those procedures; she gets diagnosed with a sprain strain and given a prescription of pain pills and released to return home. Pain continues without relief so her daughter finds me via internet and makes an appointment for her mother. Wilma shows up with her son whom was assisting her every move. She was really in pain and slouched way forward, poor woman, I even prayed for her. X-rays were taken and a lumbar 4 compression fracture was evident on X-ray. This appeared to be a new fracture, which was missed by the hospital. I prescribed some much needed bed rest, back brace, ice as needed and moist heat to increase blood circulation. I told her what positions to avoid and helpful get up and down tips to minimize her pain. I also asked her to pick up some multiple minerals due to the loss of bone density visible on her radiographic films. This type of compression fracture will heal on its own in approximately four to six months.

She was thankful I found the cause of her excruciating pain when others missed it and that I knew enough not to touch that fracture and/or when to refer out to other health care professionals as needed in this case.

Lieutenant Mike: A retired police officer in his 60's was referred to me because he was suffering from a frozen shoulder. An MRI was taken that revealed zero cause so the surgeon suggested that he shave the humerous ball and socket joint down to a smaller size to make more room for the area to pivot within the ball and socket joint that exists in the shoulder region. The surgeon also said that he would be in a sling for 6 months and 18 months of rehabilitation would be needed, and also that there was no guarantee in regards to any results. Mike was desperate and agreed. Thankfully Heidi said, please go to my chiropractor Dr. Trigo first and get a second opinion. Mike showed up on a Monday and the surgery was scheduled on that Thursday of the same week. I only had 4 days to prove to Mike that chiropractic can help him, so I asked him to come in daily and if he was approximately 25 percent better would you cancel the surgery? He said yes. I reminded him that if this doesn't work, you can always reschedule the surgery and that he had nothing to lose, he totally agreed. X-rays revealed a chronic subluxation at the C5–6 level with degeneration of the disc, stenosis and some spur growth. I let him know that the crushed nerves at the C5 and C6 level were the ones that were causing the weakening of his shoulder muscles to the point of him not even being able to lift the weight of his arm. Corrective adjustments started immediately and by day 4 he was 60 percent improved, he could raise his arm up to the level slightly above the height of his shoulder, and to my greatest joy, he canceled the surgery. Today Mike and his wife Teri are great patients under wellness care at a frequency of 2/month and he obtained full range of motion back into his shoulder at the approximately ten to twelfth visit. God bless chiropractic, we saved another life and canceled another surgery to the benefit of what was best for the patient. I love when educated patients recruit their friends and loved ones in for care.

Angela's Story: Just before I graduated from Cleveland Chiropractic College Los Angeles Aug 1999, I was dating a gal named Angela. What a singer and dancer she was, met her in a nightclub—Don't date girls that you meet in night clubs—lol. Regardless I found out later that this 25 year old lady had interstitial cystitis (burning urination with no volume, screaming pain) endometriosis, and disabling migraine headaches. Vicodin, imitrex and cocktails of fizzy drinks that lowered acidity were her daily ritual. I asked if I could adjust her to help here with her headaches, she said yes please. I started working on her spine from top to bottom. I was not surprised that her migraines went away but what I didn't expect was the many other miracles that happened to her. All her symptoms went away. She got her life back and detoxed off all her meds. She even put on some much needed weight and muscle mass. She is strong, drug/medication free still to this day and thriving.

Pastor and Wife with Baby: I was adjusting a couple when they asked me how soon after birth can you adjust a child. I replied the sooner the better. The birthing process is very traumatic for both mother and baby. Then they asked can you please check our daughter she seems to be always looking to her left and we are concerned. She was 5 weeks old, and after the realignment technique I like to use for babies, she immediately opened her eyes brighter and turned her neck to her right. Parents and I both witnessed the results right before our eyes. Success!

Christine's Story: My accountant's wife, a nurse in her 60's, came in for chiropractic care as a last ditch effort to save her from the surgeon's knife. She presented with a walker and slow steady shuffle foot drag as she walked in. This sweet lady was on many prescription medications and these took a toll on her energy levels and caused her to be very slow in her response time when asked questions. She suffered from chronic low back pain that had her hunched over, dizziness, headaches, numbness in her extremities and more. Orthopedic exam and X-rays revealed nerve impingements, Lumbar 4 and 5 were really dislodged on her. Adjustment began, her spine was not only in a posterior position but there was rotation and wedging present as well. In other words all axis of the xyz plane were present in her subluxation pattern. I call this a posterior left superior vector or PLS in regards to her L4–5. This is why X-rays are so important, not only to rule out pathology (cancer, tumors, fractures, etc.) but to be able to really zero in on correction versus guesswork. Tough case, it took 2 months at 3 times a week, and she never quit! I commended her for her persistence in following my best recommendations and never giving up hope. I had faith in the chiropractic healing powers and so did she; it definitely takes two people on the same page for results like these. She was able to lose the walker after a month and switched to a cane. At the approximate 2 month mark no more cane was needed and dizziness was also cured. No more headaches, vertigo or back ache. In fact her husband Ron no longer has to drive here everywhere and carry things for her, she is back on the move again and he now has a hard time keeping up with her! The lesson learned here is that healing takes time, and everyone is different. Remember the process always works when accurate and gentle corrective adjustments are given. Christine recently had a TMJ problem that prevented her from eating and her jaw hurt so bad that it kept her up all night. Ron called me and asked if an adjustment could help her or should I take her to the hospital? My reply was to bring her in ASAP! One adjustment in the C1-2 region and her TMJ was fixed. One adjustment, wow, another chiropractic success story.

Molly the Dog: I was on a family outing at mile square park in the city of Fountain Valley, a great place to live, when my family members went over to pet a dog. Sharon was walking her dog and we all noticed that it had a limp. We asked what happened to this small dog, Molly, that caused it to have a limp, and we were informed that jumping off the tail gate did it. I told her that I would love the opportunity to adjust the dog, and she was grateful that someone gave her a glimmer of hope besides what was offered elsewhere, surgery. Sharon brought Molly in and I used an activator adjusting tool on the dog. Molly's limp disappeared and much to my surprise, many of Sharon's family members became patients including Ben the son who still comes in today. God used Molly and I to spread the healing in our community and because of chiropractic, our great city is a healthier place to live. If Molly could speak she would bark a sincere thank you for giving her a spring back into her step.

Molly the Patient: This sweet gal has had problems getting pregnant and really wanted to be a mother and have her own child. Molly came to me for chronic headaches, neck pain and back pain. Quickly she learned how the nerves control every function in the human body. She understood that even her female reproductive system was dependent on proper nervous system function. After examination and X-rays were taken, subluxations were shown to exists at the upper cervical level (cause of her headaches) and lower 3 lumbar bones, female reproductive system function and more. I started adjusting Molly over the next few months at a frequency of 2/month due to distance she needed to drive to come see me, approx. Thirty miles. I hoped to see her weekly but I was at least happy she never went more than two to three weeks without care. Included in the education process was information pertaining to the most effective times to be active in regards to maximizing her potential to get pregnant. I revealed to her information regarding her monthly cycle, Day 1 is the start of menstruation. Day 5 is the end. Day 14 is ovulation, a day that your body is 1 degree hotter, cramping on one of your sides (egg being released from the ovary), increased desires of affection on that day, etc. On day 27 if not pregnant, blood supply is cut off to a nest that was growing, needed for the future attraction of an embryo if conception took place. Twenty-eighth day menstruation begins and the cycle starts over again. Sperm can live in the female body for forty-eight hours. So day 12–16 is the window of procreation and all the other days are for recreation. The man needs to go into this window with a high volume of sperm so three to four days prior, no ejaculation is recommended, this will assure maximum volume and high sperm count for the active 4 day window.

> ### In regards to the window of pregnancy, day 12–16 is for procreation and all the other days are for recreation! (Jeff Trigo, DC)

Molly and her friend Robyn came in the other day and I saw her pregnancy glow the minute she walked in. Smiling from ear to ear, Molly said," guess what Dr. Trigo? You got me pregnant!" I said at the front desk in front of the waiting room and office personal, no way it wasn't me! LOL It was your husband and chiropractic! I was never there, LOL! We have a lot of fun at the wellness center. She always had what it took to have a child, we just needed to remove the distortion and maximize the timing. Surprise, we have another chiropractic baby due because of the increased communication and the highways being restored and reconnected via the all mighty adjustments! Dimmer switch removed. In the time needed to prepare this book, Cross, a healthy boy, was born.

Matt the Carpenter: Imagine a man that builds stuff out of wood not being able to feel his hands! This is his livelihood, a wood working carpenter with what was said to be carpal tunnel, no longer able to provide for himself a decent living because he has lost power and feeling in his hands! MD's wanted to cut the band (flexor retinaculum) that supports all the tendons and aids in grip strength. They said this would give the carpal nerve more room! I have always been shocked at the stupidity of this suggestion. Carpal tunnel has and will always be a double crush injury. In other words, at least 2 areas of nerve must have a compression and/or squeezing pressure somewhere along the nerve for it to go numb and lose feeling. I removed the subluxation at the C7, first site, and gave him some pectoralis minor stretches to do at home; Nerve travels under this muscle as it goes into arm, and swiftly the feeling and power came back. I believe his results were fast because he gets checked semi-regularly and a lot of time didn't go by with prolonged nerve pressure therefore limiting the damage and reducing the healing time needed. He was also able to lift the heavy doors again because the sharp shooting rib pain is now absent. As a side effect of the full spine checkups, the suffering from allergies and chronic sinusitis has also disappeared. Matt's new story was telling my front desk all about how much pain his feet are always in. What the foot doctors are telling him to do, etc. I overheard this conversation and asked him to please step in my office so that I can reeducate you. I went on and told him that you have 26 bones in your feet and that one to a few of them could be out of place. Foot arches need to be maintained. We need to consider the tension on the muscles, tendons and ligaments, etc. I really tried to let him know that doctors of chiropractic spend more time in school studying human anatomy and biomechanics than any other doctor out there, and this education included the treatment necessary for proper foot care. There is also the component of VSC affecting the nerves from the low back and his regular chronic reoccurring lumbar subluxations may be the possible source of your foot pain and healing takes time. Then I said, please tell me if there is something bothering you that I may need to take a deeper look at, not the front desk. Have faith in chiropractic, it has never let you down before. Don't let this good news go in one ear and then forget as soon as you step outside of my office. Adjustments started on both of his feet. I found dropped metatarsals in both feet, dislodged talo-fibular joints, tight calf's, tight piriformis, etc. Now even his feet feel great! I see Matthew once a week, he has only wellness stories now, and refers patients often. He understands the importance of regular chiropractic care. After a few education attempts, he finally had his "A-Ha" moment of clarity with understanding regarding the maintenance of spinal health. Proactive prevention at its best demonstrated here.

"Great health is an inside job that starts with the spine. Make chiropractic part of your life. Get adjusted! Call a chiropractor today to get started on your wellness journey."
(Jeff Trigo, DC)

Pamm's Story: This sweet lady had her whole family under chiropractic care, and they were obtaining great results. The younger kids no longer had ear infections and her husband's back pain was gone and he was back earning for the family. Pamm's migraines went away, etc. However one day she came in and was very distraught. She had visited her family MD who tried to label her with the condition called fibromyalgia because of her multiple shooting neurological symptoms. She had tears in her eyes as she explained her symptoms to me. Now these shooting nerve patterns seemed to be everywhere and did not follow the normal nerve root distribution (dermatomes) along the skin pathways. So the first thing that came to my mind was B vitamins. I asked her if she was taking B vitamins. She replied that she had been taking a B complex that was prescribed to her recently for some energy loss that she was experiencing. I asked her to go home and read the labels of these B supplements and check to see if the levels were close to 100 percent USRDA, or if they were much higher. If too much B vitamins are being consumed, the side effects could be exactly what you're experiencing now, with these many shooting nerve pains (polyneuralgia). Three days went by and on her next appointment she was happy to report that it had been 2 days without these crazy shooting nerve symptoms. Her B vitamins were 2000 percent of the USRDA and even more in some cases, so she was definitely consuming toxic levels and when she quit taking them, the symptoms immediately went away; 95 percent of all Medical schools have no nutritional education program therefore how can they understand the natural ways that food can heal, or the proper levels needed for supplementation?

Uncle Angelo a.k.a. Mr. P: Angelo always believed in eating healthy, walking and taking care of his spine. My father was taking care of Mr. P's spine long before it was my turn to carry the torch. Today at 92, he is strong, can walk without assistance and his mind is as sharp as ever. Sure he loves his naps but wow what an example of the compound effect in a real life health application. At times when he is dehydrated and sipping too much espresso and red wine, his blood pressure goes way up because of low blood volume. To resolve this issue we add hydration and deep breathing inhalation exercises. Afterwards, the blood pressure was rechecked and we all witnessed a drop in blood pressure right before our eyes. When we took some new X-rays recently, I saw that upper neck brain stem pressure was present as C1–2 was totally rotated via radiographic films. After adjusting him, balance returned and energy spiked. This adjustment has had a long lasting expression of an increased in power and energy that he continues to show and now he is back on a weekly regiment of chiropractic care once again. He is active in his walking again and continues to eat healthy. I am hopeful to see him hit the 100-year mark!

10,000 Times: I can't count the number of times that a patient said something positive immediately after receiving that spinal correction. Statements like, "I can breathe again," "my sinus just opened," "now that feels so much better," "wow I don't feel the pain anymore doctor," "I can feel the pressure leaving my head," "I can put weight on my leg again," etc. It is all truth and not exaggeration! They like to tell me that I've healed them or fixed them, etc. I always reply: that the adjustment turns the power to heal back on and that the body heals itself. Amen. I ask them to tell others! I can't do this alone, I need your help and please write a testimonial online! Yelp it, Google it, Facebook it, where ever you want, just tell the story so others can benefit too.

Did I heal these any of wonderful awesome patients of mine? The answer is no. God used me as a healing tool for, His purposes, so that His Saints might truly thrive, subluxation-free again. I turned the spinal circuit breaker switch back into the "on position" and the home started to operate at full power again. The home was prewired for optimal function. Just as if a car were on a hose and the plant started to show symptoms of loss of growth, when we remove the car off the hose, the water reaches the plant, we see it start to thrive again. I can't make the plant grow; it does that all by itself! I removed the interference by adjusting the spinal vertebrae off the nerve and set forth in action what was divinely already imbedded in our genetic make-up at birth, innate wisdom. We must remember that life produces VSC, therefore don't let spinal health and maintenance fall off your appointment radar.

The observation of the compound effect can be seen here. The sooner you get that locked segment of the spine adjusted, VSC, the less damage and decay can infiltrate the surrounding areas; minimizing the time of exposure that VSC crushes the nerves and creates loss of normal joint motion thus minimizing its damaging effects. VSC sets in motion a whole cascade of symptoms fooling the best doctors into a lessor diagnosis (symptom) instead of locating and removing the cause (subluxation).

Dr. Robert Trigo Cradle Cap Kid: My pop graduated Cleveland Chiropractic College in 1967. He opened a practice in Buena Park and helped thousands of people over many years. One day he was treating a lady who left a young boy in the front lobby, he was about eight to ten years old. My dad noticed that this kid had a cheesy thick substance all over his head, known as cradle cap. This can be common in the newborns but a young boy? My dad asked the mother what was the deal with this boy of hers? She replied that she has been to many doctors and that they have prescribed many pills, potions, lotions and creams, all having no results on this embarrassing condition. My father asked, "may I please have some time with him'? The mother was thrilled and quickly responded yes please. Behind the scenes, Dr. Trigo Sr. sent a staff member to the local store to purchase

2 large bottles of Listerine. He called the child back and asked him if he would like to get rid of that stuff on the top of his head, he replied in a shy way yes. My dad soaked a towel full of Listerine and wrapped his head with it. He then left the room to adjust other patients and gave the boy some time. In the back room there were some old school X-ray development tanks and a sink. He scrubbed the kids head with a brush and then soaked a new towel and put it back on the kids head. He went back to the treatment rooms adjusting his regular flow of patients. After a second scrubbing, 45 minutes later, his head became pink and clean. No more cradle cap! 20 years later that same kid saw my dad at a relicensing seminar, and approached him while asking, are you Dr. Robert Trigo? My dad replied yes, who is asking? I am the kid that had cradle cap cured in your office 20 years ago. I'm a chiropractor now because of you! WOW. You never know how far reaching the actions or words done or said today, will echo into eternity affecting the lives of countless others tomorrow.

Dr. Robert Trigo and the woman from Japan in the wheelchair: As God is my witness; My Father in Heaven used my father on earth to heal a woman in 1989/90 in Las Vegas, during a chiropractic educational seminar provided between USA and Japan companies. She was in a wheel chair due to some injury that caused her spine to lock up with one facet climbing up and over another facet. Dr. Trigo asked my brother Greg and I to rub the myospasms and relax a certain region of her spine in order for him to accomplish a particular technique to apply on this ladies spine. After the adjustment she made a loud yell. My dad held the pressure on her spine for a few seconds, Paused, and let go.

People were gathered around; it was in a teaching environment, so there were many witnesses present. The very next day the woman who had been in a wheel chair for 10 years was up walking with assistance of her husband and a cane. Day 2 she was walking around with no cane! She slow danced on day 3, and all of us at the farewell party located in the ballroom of the Tropicana Casino, NV, watched in amazement at the wonderful power the healing adjustment has to offer those who need it.

Dr. Robert Trigo and 2 MD's with nurse, knocking on back door:
The people who knew my dad well called him Rocky, and when he
heard a soft knocking on his clinic back door, he answered it personally. To his surprise stood two MDs and a nurse looking at him with
great anticipation. This nurse had fallen on her face, dislodged her
jaw, appeared all swollen with discoloration and needed help standing
due to the medication they had her doped up with. The MDs failed
in trying to fix this, so they gave up and were knocking on the back
door, why not the front door? Chapter 7 will shed some light on this.

Rocky iced her up, doubled gripped her mandible (jaw) from
underneath, pulled it apart while realigning it and set it back into its
normal position. The MDs asked my dad how he did it and my dad
looked at them and only said, "Chiropractic" and escorted them out.
He fixed her and no thank you letter, no payment, no box of goodies,
bottle of wine nothing. He had a big heart, a servant's heart and that is
what takes to make it in our awesome profession today, passion, personality, adjusting skills, and a big heart. Don't worry about the money
it will take care of itself. Give the patient the best adjustment possible
and get out of the way of their healing. Always expect miracles when
given a chiropractic adjustment because God doesn't make junk!

"WHEN LOVE AND SKILL WORK TOGETHER, EXPECT A MASTERPIECE." (B. J. PALMER)

It's an absolute privlidge to be a chiropractor and public servant
for healing. I wish I could write more testimonials and document the
many other healing miracles that happened with the chiropracTIC
adjustment. You should know that miracles are happening all over
the world in many chiropractic clinicls worldwide, so please don't fill
that prescription and swallow the lies.

No longer will you be a pill popper and act in an unscientific
way, get adjusted and return proper nervous system function to your
master system instead, this also restores joint motion, reversing arthritis, and stopping arthritis in its tracks. Today's challenge... Make an
appointment to get checked for VSC. You too should enjoy the heal-

ing that follows the adjustment and wellness lifestyles. It's not where you have been but where you are going that matters. Feeling good gets addictive, and that is a good thing to always want, so what are you waiting for, have zero lag time! Every spine matters, the sooner the better, minimize the damage of VSC.

I hope you enjoyed reading about these awesome people who found extrodinary healing. It is a great and wonderful feeling to know that our body has its very own built in healing powers. We just need the right stuff! Chiropractic adjustments, real wholesome nutitional intake and plenty of regular exercise are the long term fundamental keys to reach the 100 year milestone. There are so many different ways to adjust subluxations and some techniques work better than others. I encourage you to keep trying and never give up when it comes to your health and wellness. Teaching chiropractic technique gave me a full bag of tricks that I discovered is really necessary for amazing results. Some techniques work great on one person but not on the other, so as I said, it's paramount to have a plethora of tools in your adjusting repertoire.

"Once a week, it has got to be" (Debbie Satriano), a long term patient in regards to her feeling the best she could be.

"Dr. Trigo, in all the many years you have adjusted me, you have never hurt me and I want you to know how wonderful and skilled I think you are" Tom Vasil, age 70+

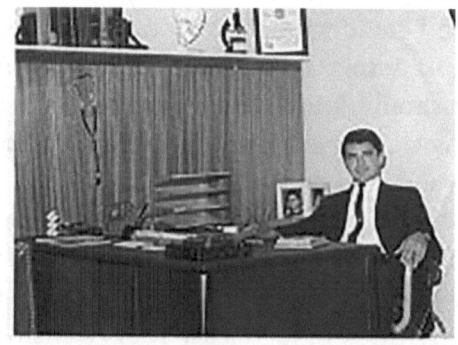

Dr. Robert F.S. Trigo, D.C. 1970's

CHAPTER 7

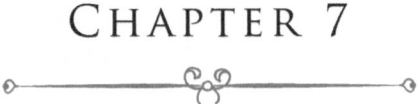

Against All Odds

Chiropractic has been under assault ever since that deaf man named Harvey Lillard received his first adjustment on September 18, 1895 by a man named Daniel David Palmer, a.k.a. D.D. Palmer.

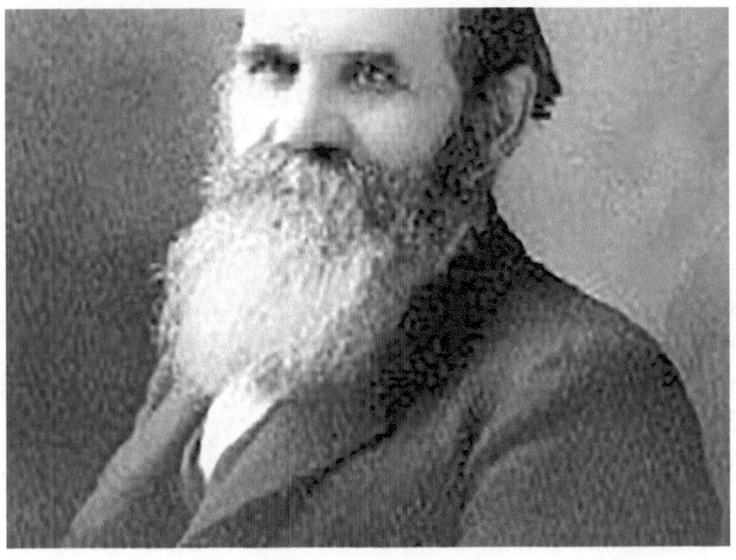

The righteous man walks in his integrity; His children are blessed after him. (Proverbs 20:7 NKJV)

Lillard's hearing was restored and after the adjustment said "I can hear the wagon wheels in the street", the medical field a.k.a. American Medical Association, tried to eliminate a competitor and spread misconceptions about this wonderful new found scientific breakthrough. It seems that there is no money or profit in curing dis/ease therefore sickness care becomes big business in America even today!

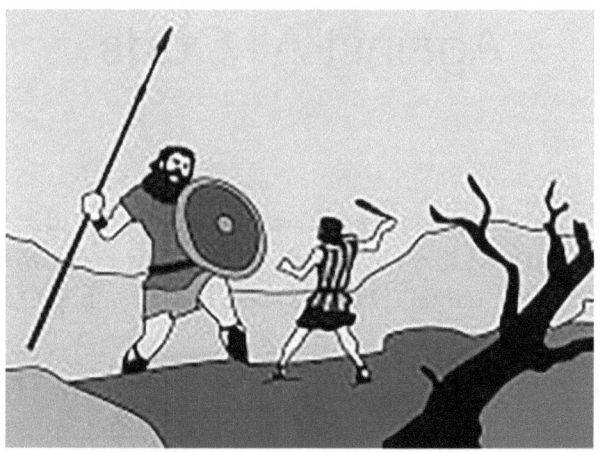

The MD and PhDs, needs to admit that subluxations exist! People find a public healer nearby, a.k.a. chiropractor, and get checked for subluxations. Do this first and not as a last result! The chiropractor will examine your spine, do orthopedic, neurological and muscle tests as needed, take X-rays (if necessary), and with palpation and gentle corrective specific care, start fixing the bent frame and its subluxations. The sooner we start caring for our spine the sooner we obtain wellness. Adjustments to the spine, a natural diet and regular exercise implemented at the youngest age possible will yield maximum compounded health effects. Calling out all doctors, the best recommendation for the patient must be considered for their wellbeing! Patient, have you heard all options? When a light accurate gentle realignment is given to correct subluxation expect miracles. This must be considered first not last when giving the patient a best recommendations. I often hear people advising against chiropractic care and that is totally insane. That's like listening to someone telling you to stop brushing your teeth or don't work out! This is totally ludicrous. Stop the Madness! Use the information in this book to decide what are the best options for you and your family. The best non-invasive holistic natural results with a proven track record to create happy patients willing to write a testimonial in regards to their return to wellness absent of dis/ease. Only chiropractors have hundreds of happy healthy patients writing testimonials.

Adjust The Spine First, Not Last!
You'll save thousands of dollars and live well.
(Jeffrey Trigo, DC)

"Adjust your Thots" Ask the right questions, for example, is my master system turned to an off position? Am I subluxated? Is this arthritis pain I feel because I have lost normal joint motion? A pinched nerve will cause my life force to be altered or diminished therefore stop chasing the symptoms and locate the cause. These pinched nerves can cause so many symptoms fooling the best doctors because they are not looking for subluxation therefore missing cause and treating the symptoms with poor results and harmful side effects. Get Adjusted World.

To not recommend the best options to a patient seeking care from a physician is absolute negligence. Adjustments should always be recommended even with co-management in which the MD and DC work together to help the patient obtain the fastest safest long lasting best results as possible for the patient's wellbeing. Otherwise this goes against the Chiropractic and Hippocratic Oath, which in short means 'to do no harm' and be the best doctor you can be. It's for the publics own good.

Chiropractic Oath via Texas Chiropractic College (TCC)

I do hereby affirm before God and assembled witnesses that I will keep this oath and stipulation:

To hold in esteem and respect those who taught me this chiropractic healing art; to follow the methods of treatment which according to my ability and judgement I consider for the benefit of my patients; to abstain from whatever is deleterious and mischievous, to stand ready at all times to serve my fellow man without distinction of race, creed or color.

With purity I will pass my life and practice my art; I will at all times consider the patients under my care as of supreme importance, I will not spare myself in rendering them the help which I have been taught to give by my alma matter; I will keep inviolate all things revealed to me as a physician.

While I continue this oath inviolate, may it be granted to me to enjoy life and the practice of chiropractic healing art, respected by all men at all times.

Hippocratic Oath:

I swear by Apollo the physician, and Aesculapius, and Health, and All-heal, and all the gods and goddesses, that, according to my ability and judgment, I will keep this Oath and this stipulation—to reckon him who taught me this Art equally dear to me as my parents, to share my substance with him, and relieve his necessities if required; to look upon his offspring in the same footing as my own brothers, and to teach them this Art, if they shall wish to learn it, without fee or stipulation; and that by precept, lecture, and every other mode of instruction, I will impart a knowledge of the Art to my own sons, and those of my teachers, and to disciples bound by a stipulation and oath according to the law of medicine, but to none others. I will follow that system of regimen which, according to my ability and judgment, I consider for the benefit of my patients, and abstain from whatever is deleterious and mischievous. I will give no deadly medicine to any one if asked, nor suggest any such counsel; and in like manner I will not give to a woman a pessary to produce abortion. With purity and with holiness I will pass my life and practice my Art. I will not cut persons laboring under the stone, but will leave this to be done by men who are practitioners of this work. Into whatever houses I enter, I will go into them for the benefit of the sick, and will abstain from every voluntary act of mischief and corruption; and, further from the seduction of females or males, of freemen and slaves. Whatever, in connection with my professional practice or not, in connection with it, I see or hear, in the life of men, which ought not to be spoken of abroad, I will not divulge, as reckoning that all such should be kept secret. While I continue to keep this Oath unviolated, may it be granted to me to enjoy life and the practice of the art, respected by all men, in all times! But should I trespass and violate this Oath, may the reverse be my lot!

I want to make a few points here:

1. In summary, "do no harm", however when a surgeon recommends an invasive surgery without first trying chiropractic is absolute insanity and harm to the people. Wake up America this is not ok!

2. Getting a patient addicted to pain pills and opioids instead of checking for subluxation, which can always lead to chronic pain syndromes, is irresponsible and a shame. The physician failed to find the cause and chose to mask it with pill popping unleashing what will soon be a cascade of side effects to bank on.

3. Apollo and Aesculapius? There is only one God, and He exists in 3 unique different individuals yet 3 in 1. A great mystery the awesome Trinity of God: Father, Son and Holy Spirit.

"I am the God of Abraham, the God of Isaac and the God of Jacob? God is not the God of the dead, but of the living." (Matthew 22:23)

You may have heard that "couples that pray together, stay together," well, contemplate this: "couples that get adjusted together age well together" Jeff Trigo, D.C.

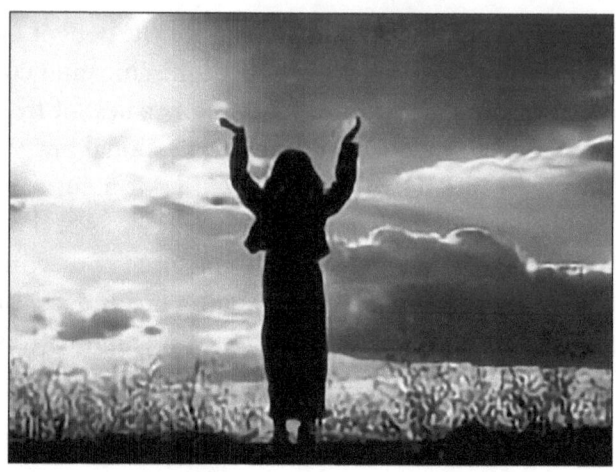

"You shall love the Lord your God with all of your heart, with all your soul, and with all your strength." (Deuteronomy 6:5)

When the vertebral body has been dislodged due to chemical, emotional or physical force, this reduces the exit site of the canal space for the pathway of the spinal nerve. This condition is usually diagnosed as stenosis if viewed from the side with imaging techniques. Adjust the bone forward versus recommending a laminectomy, which cuts bone away to make a hole larger for the nerve when a gentle adjustment does the same thing; makes the canal larger! One adjustment is approximately $50 bucks while the other procedure starts in the 10's of thousands, causing fusion and harms the patients, this is total malpractice and should absolutely be a last resort, not the first. As a last resort I mean that the patient has tried at least 4 different chiropractors. New flash, disc can heal too.

The "Quack" Label

It took an antitrust lawsuit filed against the American Medical Association (AMA) in 1976 to reveal the magnitude of the scope of their plan which was to eliminate the Chiropractic profession as a whole because they felt threatened by its mere existence. Regular slander of the chiropractic profession with constant verbal bashing had been taking place on a regular basis. It was said to have no association with the Chiropractor and to call them "quacks." Fight that they get no insurance pay and threaten the hospitals to do no business with them if they work with chiropractors, etc. This went on for a century!

Chiropractors had to fight for their survival and to get the recognition that is due to them. The Doctor of Chiropractic now occupies positions in the military, hospitals and professional sports teams, besides the family chiropractor doctor. Well this has not always been the chiropractor's case. The medical doctors who were slandering the profession of chiropractic maintained that this new science was unscientific and unethical, but yet in fact the dispensing of drugs was actually more unscientific and dangerous versus its competitor, the chiropractic profession which was receiving results that they could never obtain. Chiropractic as a whole stayed separate and never joined the AMA maintaining a holistic position of a naturopath and homeopathic healer. It was found by many authors in the mid 1800's that the AMA's intent was not to protect the public from unethical chiropractors but was to decrease competition for financial gain. By convincing lawmakers and state legislators with their big profit revenues that came from cheap drugs and big income, that their profession was the only one that was scientific, all other doctors were singled out and the AMA thrived for the next 100 plus years as they got endorsed by everyone. Believe it or not this is still happening today with the vaccination and immunization scams and scandals. Big Pharma controls congress and makes sure certain laws can pass that ensure big profits but not big health in any way shape or form.

When a nonbeliever sins he is breaking God's law. When a believer sins he is breaking God's heart. We have nothing to offer God, therefor be humble and obedient to His laws, they are for our own good. Teach me oh Lord all your ways so that I may live in truth and love always, in Jesus name I pray, amen.

D. D. Palmer founded the first chiropractic college in America, located in Davenport Iowa in the year 1897. He called it Palmer

College of Chiropractic. D. D. Palmer had a son and his name was Bartlett Joshua Palmer, DC, a.k.a. B. J. Palmer and he was the main promoter of the profession of chiropractic.

D. D. Palmer had proclaimend that chiropractic care was for multiple cures therefore being looked upon as a menace by the drug dispensers and medical authorities. Palmer taught that we had an inner healer of innate wisdom which governed health and that rather than receive medical treatments, adjustments were warrented instead to restore communiction of the neuro-pathways being the perfered treatment of choice.

Chiropractors then started to get arrested for practicing medicine without a license with the first arrest being in 1905 to chiropractor E. J. Whipple and G. W. Johnson, they were convicted and served jail time for adjusting spines. D. D. Palmer also spent twenty-three days in the Scott Couty Jail in Iowa for the same offense. The need for a chiropractic joint defense team (Universal Chiropractors Association) was then established in 1906 to help those being prosecuted for adjusting the spine and "practicing medicine without a license."

In 1907 a victory was celebrated when Wisconsin versus Morikubo, a chiropractor arrested for practicing osteopathy and medicine without a license, challanged the precedent set in the Whipple and Johnson case. This resulted in a legal establishment of chiropractic as a separate and distinct profession from medicine and osteopathy based largely on the chiropractic philosophy.

Despite a legal precedent which allowed the chiropractor to adjust the spine, some shy of 700 more chiropractors would be arrested and do time for practicing medicine without a license in which at that time most states did not offer chiropractic licenses because they didn't exist yet therefore establishing our great professions next legal victory. In 1913 Kansas became the first state to establish a separate chiropractic board and 100 percent legalize the practice of chiropractic. By the 1920s half the country had similar laws and licensure in place with the last state being Louisiana in 1974. Regardless of this legal precedent that was shaping America into a pro chiropractic arena, the AMA continued to wage ongoing campaigns against the art and science of chiropractic calling us unscientific, quacks, charlatans, snake oil peddelers, and an out right "cult." In the 1929–1950 state test included surgical procedures in which chiropractors do not perform therefore making it very difficult to pass the exam and shrinking the number of licensed chiropractors while increasing the number of unlicensed doctors practicing anyways and being subjected to arrest. In 1963 the AMA formed "The Committee on Quackery" and said that rabid dogs and chiropractors fall into the same category, and chiropractors were nice but that they killed people. Around the same time 1962–1963, under the leadership of Robert B. Throckmorton, the AMA adopted the so-called "Iowa Plan" which was to cause a containment of the chiropractic profession, causing a decline in popularity and action steps in this plan to encourage ethical complaints against the doctor of chiropractic. The action steps also included a disunity amongst chiropractors and impose unfair reimbursements with health insurance plans while blocking any hospital affiliations. Talk about a desperate AMA that definitely doesn't have the public's best health or interest in mind, ever! It is all about the money! In 1976 during the trial of Chester C. Wilk versus AMA, hundreds of thousands of documents trying to discredit chiropractic was brought up in court. Including AMA ghost writers for TV and newspapers with the goal of tarnishing the chiropractors reputation in the public eye. Even guidance counselors for schools were being bribed by the AMA not to mention chiropractic careers to upcoming college kids interested in health professions.

Three lawsuits were settled over the next dozen years, and the AMA relaxed its position on the referral of patients to chiropractors by medical doctors. In 1980 the AMA changed its policy in its Principles of Medical Ethics documents to reflect allowing the patient to choose which doctor they wanted to see, to be refered to, or be treated by. In 1987 US District Judge Susan Getzendanner found the AMA and its codefendants guilty in violation of the Sherman Antitrust Act. In this verdict the Judge ruled that the AMA decided to contain and eliminate chiropractic as a profession and that it was the AMA's intent "to destroy a competitor."

As the years went by, some old bad habits never die as some MDs continued to tell the patient not to see a chiropractor. In whole the current status, chiropractic is much more widely accepted and co-management of patients is much more popular since the turn of the century. Chiropractors despite all odds continue to get results that medication just can't obtain and now DCs serve alongside the military, co-manage with medical practitioners in clinics and hospitals all throughout the United States and are becoming more and more the go-to doctor of choice because of the quick safe relief patients are regularly obtaining.

"One man tells a lie, dozens repeat it as truth."
(Chinese Proverb)

When I was attending Cleveland Chiropractic College Los Angeles, before the turn of the century, I remember learning about studies and research that resulted in favorable proof that the chiropractic methods were superior to its counterpart MD methods and their outside in thinking and flawed ideology. Many studies come to mind and I look forward to discussing some of them with you. Remember this, the adjustment results are always much more favorable, when subluxation is removed, versus pain management, scalpels and screws which ignore causation.

The Windsor Autopsies:
Dr. Henry Winsor MD, a doctor from the Philadelphia area, showed interest when he observed that the chiropractic adjustment, unlocking vertebral subluxation, repeatedly got rid of various diseases amongst many case studies, therefore causing him to become intrigued and seek more evidence. He asked himself how these adjustments are yielding such great results despite not giving them any drugs or surgery. So he planned a unique experiment that would examine and dissect the human cadaver along with various other vertebrates and see if there was a correlation between subluxation (cause) and disease (effect). In a cadaver finding subluxation is more difficult due to rigormortis (whole body stiffness) and you can't ask

the person when you push gently on each spinal level, does it hurt here? Etc. So what he decided to do was to look for the long term side effects of subluxation: Degenerative disc, osteophytes and spurs, stenosis, nerve interference, misaligned vertebra and abnormal curves on the spine, etc.

He conducted his spinal dissections autopsies on approximately 75 humans and 22 cat cadavers at the University of Pennsylvania and published his results in the same year in the Medical Times, Nov 1921. His findings were overwhelmingly conclusive in that maintaining a healthy spine is vital to enjoying a wellness lifestyle. Dr. Winsor was able to find 221 diseased organs and when the nerve was traced back to the spinal level in which it originated from, 212 of those levels had evidence of long term subluxation, misalignments and/ or abnormal curvatures located at the same level in which the spine exits and controls the organ while the other ten diseases were located one level above or below the actual level which is the control area for function of that organ. That is 100 percent correlation between disease of the spine, and at that level of nerve loss which controls organ function, becoming diseased and killing the individual.

> **"The disease seems to precede old age and to cause it. The spine becomes stiff first and old age follows. Therefore we may say, a man is as old as his spine..."**
> **(Dr. Henry Winsor, MD)**

The many types of diseases found throughout the body he concluded were caused by slight disruptions in the spine therefore diminishing function by irritating the sympathetic nerve ganglia causing vaso-motor spasms and diminished blood flow to adjacent organs innervated by involved nerve. This in return, caused a diminished nerve supply and blood flow to the organs, caused the organs to prematurely age, decay and die. He also mentioned that this process takes about 2 decades and could easily be avoided with proper spinal realignments and maintenance. He went on to say that spinal disease precedes disease and old age therefore making it important to have regular spinal realignments for maximum nervous system function thereby living a longer healthier life. He also witnessed reversal of disease when adjustments were implemented.

The Manga Report:

In 1993 the country of Canada conducted the largest analysis of the effectiveness of the chiropractic doctor when used as a portal of entry doctor first versus using the medical protocol. The Ontario Ministry of Health therefore recommended the management of lower back pain be moved away from the medical protocol and allow the doctor of chiropractic to become the doctor of choice due to the cost effectiveness as well as the results the patient obtained from the realignment of the vertebra. This they concluded would save the financial problems that the Canadian government was suffering due to high health care cost, while providing a means to end the disability that handicapped the patient, thus ending an epidemic of hundreds of thousands of sufferers of low back pain that would end up causing disability and morbidity pinpointing this as the most expensive cost of workers compensation cost in North America.

The Canadian Government report concluded with the following findings:

- On the evidence, particularly the most scientifically valid clinical studies, spinal manipulation applied by chiropractors is shown to be more effective than alternative treatments for low back pain. Many medical therapies are of questionable validity or are clearly inadequate;
- There is no clinical or case-control study that demonstrates or even implies that chiropractic spinal manipulation is unsafe in the treatment of low back pain. Some medical treatments are equally safe, but others are unsafe and generate iatrogenic (doctor-induced) complications for low back pain patients. Our reading of the literature suggests that chiropractic manipulation is safer than medical management of low back pain;
- Indeed, several existing medical therapies of low back pain are generally contraindicated on the basis of the existing

clinical trials. There is also some evidence in the literature to suggest that spinal manipulations are less safe and less effective when performed by non-chiropractic professionals;

- There is an overwhelming body of evidence indicating that chiropractic management of low back pain is more cost-effective than medical management;
- There would be highly significant cost savings if more management of low back pain was transferred from physicians to chiropractors. Evidence from Canada and other countries suggests potential savings of many hundreds of millions annually;
- Workers' compensation studies report that injured workers with the same specific diagnosis of low back pain returned to work much sooner when treated by chiropractors than by medical physicians;
- There is good empirical evidence that patients are very satisfied with chiropractic management of low back pain and considerably less satisfied with medical physician management;
- The use of chiropractic has grown steadily over the years and chiropractors are now accepted as a legitimate healing profession by the public and an increasing number of medical physicians;
- In our view, the following offers an overwhelming case in favor of much greater use of chiropractic services in the management of low back pain:
- The effectiveness and cost effectiveness of chiropractic management of low back pain
- The untested, questionable or harmful nature of many current medical therapies
- The economic efficiency of chiropractic care for low back pain compared with medical care
- The safety of chiropractic care
- The higher satisfaction levels expressed by patients of chiropractors.

The following recommendations were also included in the report:

- There should be a shift in policy to encourage and prefer chiropractic services for most patients with low back pain;
- Chiropractic services should be fully insured under the Ontario Health Insurance Plan;
- Chiropractic services should be fully integrated into the health care system;
- Chiropractors should be employed by tertiary hospitals in Ontario;
- Hospital privileges should be extended to all chiropractors for the purposes of treatment of their own patients who have been hospitalized for other reasons, and for access to diagnostic facilities relevant to their scope of practice and patients' needs;
- Chiropractic should have access to all pertinent patient records and tests from hospitals, physicians, and other health care professionals upon the consent of their patients;
- Since low back pain is of such significant concern to workers' compensation, chiropractors should be engaged at a senior level by Workers' Compensation Board to assess policy, procedures and treatment of workers with low back injuries;
- A very good case can be made for making chiropractors the gatekeepers for management of low back pain in the workers' compensation system in Ontario;
- The government should make the requisite research funds and resources available for further clinical evaluations of chiropractic management of low back pain, and for further socioeconomic and policy research concerning the management of low back pain generally;
- Chiropractic education in Ontario should be in the multidisciplinary atmosphere of a university with appropriate public funding;

- Finally, the government should take all reasonable steps to actively encourage cooperation between providers, particularly the chiropractic, medical and physiotherapy professions.

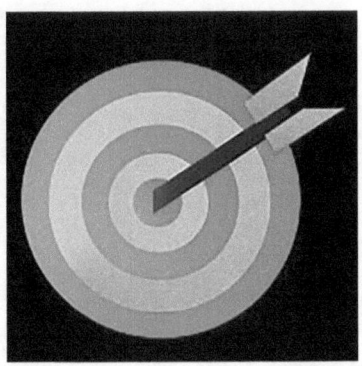

The Effectiveness and Cost Effectiveness of Chiropractic Management of Low-Back Pain (The Manga Report). Pran Manga and Associates (1993)–University of Ottawa, Canada.

New studies have proven that chiropractic adjustments at the upper cervical area are the most effective treatment for tension headaches, otitis media (ear infections) and depression. Expect more and more favorable studies to be consistently released as the cause, subluxation, is removed and function is restored naturally without medication and surgery. There will always be resistance and uneducated people that may want to tell you not to go to a chiropractor, but at these times you need to recall the facts, we all get subluxations and they can no longer be ignored. If you have had a bad experience with a chiropractic adjustment then either tell your chiropractor and have him or her do something else or change your chiropractor. Adjustments restore joint motion and nerve supply allowing the body to heal naturally, drug free and without surgical interventions. To live well, move well, eat well and think well we must add the chiropractic adjustment on a regular basis. Only with 100 percent nerve supply and joint motion can you then be considered living in the subluxation free zone, a place where thriving and fullness of life can be expressed freely.

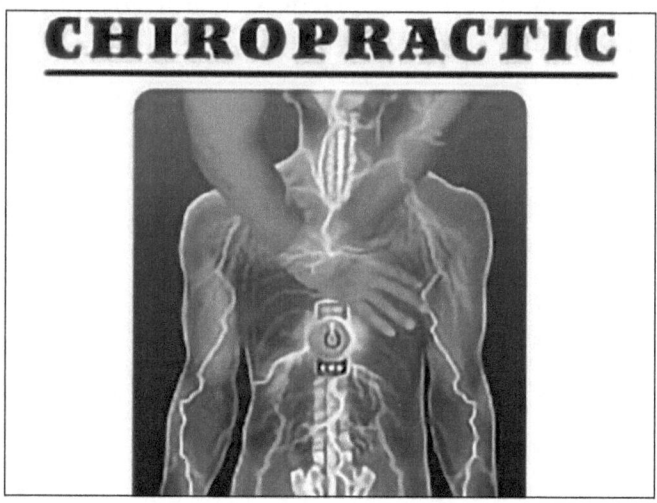

"Chiropractors do not manipulate; they do not use the process of manipulating: they adjust." (D. D. Palmer, DC)

Universal intelligence is the source of life, and the knowledge of intelligence exists everywhere. Therefore we must be intelligent in design. Innate wisdom is governed by universal intelligence and it is therefore and educated intelligence. Our body's wisdom flows through the nervous system and depends on complete unimpaired function for the expression of life and wellness.

"In the spirit we have transformation, in the flesh we have trash formation." Pastor Bert Almazan

"Pour into me, oh, God. I desire so much more of You and less of me, so empty me, cleanse me, purify me while filling me with the presence of Your Holy Spirit daily, in Jesus's name, amen." Servant of God

CHAPTER 8

Move Well

I n the neurobiological review 2007, leading researchers discovered that the brain is like a battery and it needs to be charged. That charge comes from normal movement of the spine and vigorous exercise.

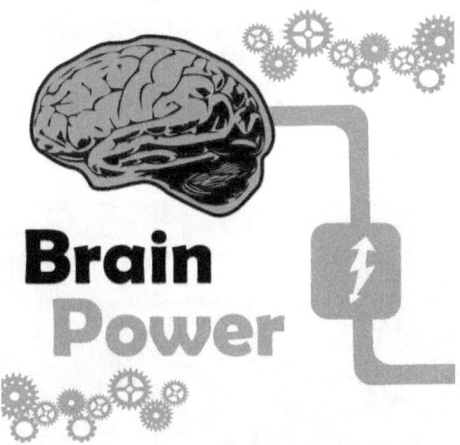

You can test this yourself when the next time you are falling asleep, get up and move around a bunch, it will wake you right up; 2007 discoveries also included what we can call energy robbers, subluxations. Locked joints bombard certain parts of the brain with noci-receptor noise on the subconscious level thus draining our battery. In other words multiple subluxations inhibit the body's ability to fully recharge during sleep therefore causing people to wake up tired and sluggish. I believe this is one of the main reasons America depends on coffee so much, everyone needs a kick start because only 10 percent of the public has a chiropractor, what a shame.

You learned in earlier chapters that movement is life to the joints thus causing the fluid lubricating and oxygen delivery system of function to perform at optimum levels which keep the disc and cartilage alive. Well in this chapter I will also be discussing the effects that exercise has on our mood, our heart function, our stamina, muscles and overall effects of wellness that it creates as we continue to move and train our body into the fine machines they were intended to be. This chapter will not teach you how to work out using proper form. That is what a personal trainer is for. Feel free to ask your trainer questions regarding exercise and learn from their expertise. This is simply a chapter on why exercise is so important and it is my wish that new habits will be created and fitness will be addicting to you and that your life, and this book, will also inspire your friends into fitness action as well, while providing a wellness education that is long overdue.

Five Types of Exercises

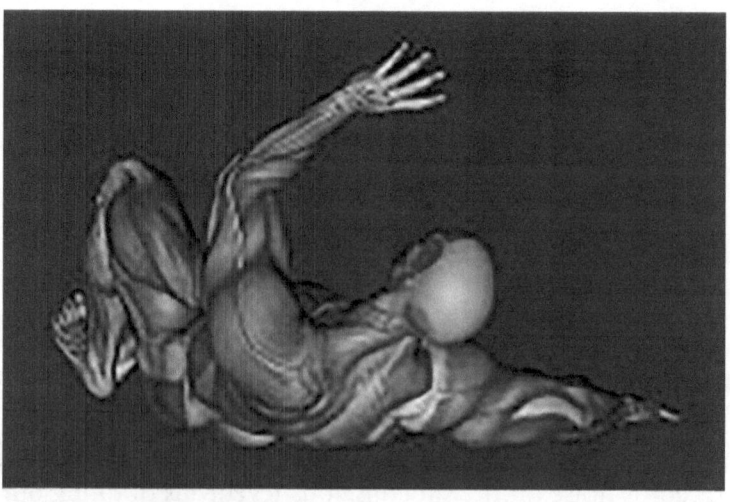

Strength Training: This type of exercise builds muscle mass and makes the muscles larger, toner and stronger. This type of exercise will help you to perform the necessary everyday strenuous activities that come along the way like climbing stairs, carrying supplies to and from the car, putting on snow chains, furniture moving, etc. This includes activities such as lifting weights, resistance bands, body weight workouts like pushups, pull ups, bar dips, sit-ups, hard runs while possibly caring extra weight, etc. After interviewing competitive lifters regarding how they achieved such great success at their body building techniques, what was revealed was besides a diet that supports muscle mass and recovery, the workout technique that yields fast results and limits injury is the following:

A. Pick only a few muscles to train and really put them through a strenuous workout. An example would be chest, triceps and abdomen, or back, shoulder and biceps. After the workout you can give that muscle groups four to five days off.

B. The right weight to start with would be one that can handle a 20–25 repetitions (Reps) and the muscle starts to burn on set 1.

C. Set 2 add weight and get 15–20 reps before the burn.

D. Set 3 add weight and get 10–15 reps before the burn.

E. Set 4 add weight and get 8–10 reps before the burn.

F. Set 5 add weight and do a burn out set, do as many as you can, then remove 30 percent of the weight, do as many as you can, remove more weight again and do as many as you can, etc. until you can barely lift the smallest weight just 3–5 times. A spotter is necessary, this person helps you take the weight off and helps you lift load off of you if muscles fail.

Endurance: This is a type of aerobic exercise that increases your cardio output and respiration. In other words it makes your heart and lungs stronger. Types of Endurance exercises are activities like hiking, jogging, participating in sports, walking, skiing, swimming, dancing, biking and other laborious jobs and various repetitive activities. I love the workout videos that are available in the market place today. They have workouts that can really make you sweat while training every muscle in your body in the comfort of your own living room.

Flexibility: Being flexible stretches your muscles and helps prevent injury while staying limber and agile. It allows you to move around easier and reduces the chance of falls, etc. All activities become a bit easier and better circulation happens in flexible regions as opposed to stuck and tight areas.

I like to stretch in my spa. That hot water really gives the muscles and tendons plenty of blood supply to limit tearing and so forth. It has been shown in a collegiate experiment in regards to stretching, that a little every day like 30 seconds daily, is more effective versus once a week for 10 minutes. Also yoga can be helpful for flexibility just be cautious of neck and back flexion because that reduces the spinal curves while adding a load of pressure on the disc. So remember the compound effect in this action, because doing it on a regular basis really reaps benefits; Daily stretching is one of many important factors to prevent injury and tears.

Balance: Exercises that help bring strength to the core and lower limbs which can aid in the prevention of falls especially in the elderly are balance exercises. Back extensions like superman's, standing on one foot, high stepping, slow movements while balancing symmetrically on one leg at a time like Tai Chi, yoga, etc. Standing on balance boards or wobble boards. Barefoot walking on the sand not only helps rub off dead skin, but will help strengthen all those tiny bone to bone connective soft tissue structures (muscles, tendons, ligaments) responsible for adding balance and stability to the top of the foot and arches of our foot, etc.

Circuit Training: This is one of the most popular types of workouts. It involves high intensity burst of energy as your workout pace remains fast and you do 30–60 seconds intervals with some short cooling down periods as you move to the next exercise station. It can offer a full body workout in 30 minutes or less and will also help with cardiovascular strength while building muscles and adding tone to them. This type of exercise will have 6–12 movements that you move through and repeat 3 times each. Circuit training will burn calories while avoiding boredom. Because you are doing movements with mostly your body, or using ropes, light weights, pullup bars, etc. Heavy weights are not being utilized thus aiding in injury prevention. Benefits are obtained within 30 minutes or less and this type of training is ideal for the person with a busy schedule.

Many exercises have multiple components of the above types of exercise combined within one activity. Like basketball, surfing, yard work, etc. Exercise will help you control your weight, keep you in a great mood due to the endorphins produced during strenuous exercise. Keeping your body in regular motion will help reduce the risk of heart disease. Exercise helps regulate blood sugar levels and manage insulin levels. If you are a smoker, exercise can help you quit. Regular exercise will also keep your mental thoughts positive, keep you learning and adapting as you age while maintaining a sharp thought process. A strong body that trains regularly and consumes the proper mineral rich diet will absolutely create stronger bones; a great benefit for the later decades in life. If you want to remain sexually active then regular exercise is essential for proper blood flow and stamina needed to perform at optimum levels. Longevity has been linked to those who exercise regularly also, so if you want to see the 80's, 90's, or even triple digits, get off the couch and move your body.

"Physical fitness takes commitment to exercise just as it requires good nutrition. But it doesn't have to be painful. Just the opposite: Vigorous exercise actually is stimulating. It boosts your energy levels, invigorates your mind, and just feels good afterwards. The hardest part, of course, is getting started." (Jack LaLanne)

Avoiding the Plateau Effect: If you keep your workouts fun and different, you will avoid the ugly plateau effect. That's a zone where you can only run the same time or distance, or stop building mass or losing weight if that's what you are training for. Just can't get over the hump and reach that goal you set for yourself? That is a plateau. People that do the same thing on a regular basis expecting different results equal insanity. One must change it up and a new exercise that the body is not used to doing to continue moving up that fitness ladder. An example of that would be: Day1 biking. Day 2 was swimming. Day 3 was weight training. Day 4 you trained a different area with weight training. Day 5 you did sit ups, pullups, and stretching. Day 6 was a golf day. On the seventh day you rested. Day 8 was a hiking exploration. Day 9 you participated in your favorite sports. Day 10 the house got cleaned. Day 11 was gardening day. Day 12 you played tennis. Day 13 weight training. Day 14 was another day of rest. Day 15 Work Out Video, etc. Change it up. Notice the one day per week of rest, even God rested on the seventh day.

"Remember the Sabbath day, to keep it holy." (Exodus 20:8)

Goal of ten thousand: It's recommended to walk at least ten thousand steps a day. Wearing a pedometer can help you track this daily goal. This endeavor is not so difficult to achieve so start off at a much lesser number, and increase gradually over time until 30 days have passed and you're at 10K. One of the best benefits of exercise is the fact that you get to fully drain your battery (energy supply) thus receiving deeper sleep during the recharging process. Make walking daily a minimum health goal and as your step count reaches the 10K mark, know that you are increasing your life span, reducing blood pressure, losing weight, helping your joints and so much more. There have been many studies on the benefits of walking, you can search them for yourself and see endless benefits. You can even walk in place, just start moving that body of yours and reap the benefits of a healthier life. Ready, Set, Go. Once you've begun you're already half done.

"Exercise to stimulate not to annihilate. The world wasn't formed in a day and neither were we. Set small goals and build upon them." (Lee Haney)

50 Benefits of Exercise:

1. Makes the heart a stronger and a more efficient pump.
2. Lowers resting heart rate.
3. Makes the lungs stronger while improving respiratory efficiency.
4. Provides more oxygen in the blood stream, important for all systems.
5. Increases metabolic rate.

"True enjoyment comes from exercise of the mind and exercise of the body; the two are ever united." (Wilhelm Von Humboldt)

6. Improves endurance and athletic performance.
7. Increases blood flow to the brain and other vital organs.
8. Helps manage blood pressure.
9. Improves overall mood and feeling of wellbeing.
10. Stimulates digestion while allowing for better elimination.

"Exercise is labor without awareness." (Samuel Johnson)

11. Eases muscle tension while aiding in circulation.
12. Increases muscle contraction capabilities while improving reaction speed.
13. Stronger muscles help hold your spine in its proper position.
14. Prevention of injury.
15. Keeps the joints and cartilage alive and lubricated.

"Movement is medicine for creating change in a person's physical, emotional and mental states." (Carol Welch)

16. Reduces the chance of chronic diseases.
17. Boost energy.
18. Increased flexibility and agility.
19. Lowers stress levels.

20. Removes lactic acid from the blood.

"Exercise and application produce order in our affairs, health of body, cheerfulness of mind, and these make us precious to our friends." (Thomas Edison)

21. Increases coordination.
22. Burns calories and causes weight loss.
23. Increased self-confidence.
24. Helps balance and maintain healthy cholesterol levels.
25. Reduces the chance of disabilities.

"We do not stop exercising because we grow old—we grow old because we stop exercising." (Kenneth Cooper)

26. Builds stronger bones.
27. Reduces the chance for stroke.
28. Reduces the chance of dementia.
29. Tones muscles and helps prevent varicose veins.
30. Reduces inflammation.

"Physical fitness in not only one of the most important keys to a healthy body, it is the basis of a dynamic and creative intellectual activity"
John F. Kennedy

31. Helps regulate proper hormone levels.
32. You feel better about yourself and can attract a mate easier.
33. Provides a way to let off steam and anger if needed.
34. Helps eliminate toxins from the body.
35. Provides a healthy way to pass the time.

"Those who think they have not time for bodily exercise will sooner or later have to find time for illness." (Edward Stanley)

36. Boost immune system function.

37. Saves you money by not paying for sickness.
38. Joint motion helps to ease and eliminates arthritic pain.
39. Can create new friends that have healthy habits also.
40. Can add years to your life, and life to your years.

"Feed your fitness. Starve your mediocrity." (Krystal Breakley)

41. Improves the quality of your life.
42. Can keep you independent as you age.
43. Burns body fat.
44. Helps to maintain healthy arteries.
45. You can eat more without gaining weight.

"Lack of activity destroys the good condition of every human being, while movement and methodical physical exercise save it and preserve it." (Plato)

46. You will be able to be sexually active longer.
47. Can prevent or manage type 2 diabetes by making insulin work better while lowering blood sugars.
48. Increased self-control and discipline.
49. Helps ones psychological functions.
50. Improves the way you see and think about yourself.

**15 minutes to warm up? Does a lion warm up when he's hungry? "Uh oh, here comes an antelope. Better warm up." No! He just goes out there and eats the sucker.
(Jack LaLanne)**

I am sure that you can come up with many more reasons for yourself, family, or career as to why you should exercise more. Just keep in mind that the compound effect will start to be observable as you stick to it. Results will be seen not just measurable on a scale, but by the quality of life gained. The work expended during physical exercise will pay off in priceless confidence and life-long dividends.

"Training gives us an outlet for suppressed energies created by stress and thus tones the spirit just as exercise conditions the body"
Arnold Schwarzenegger

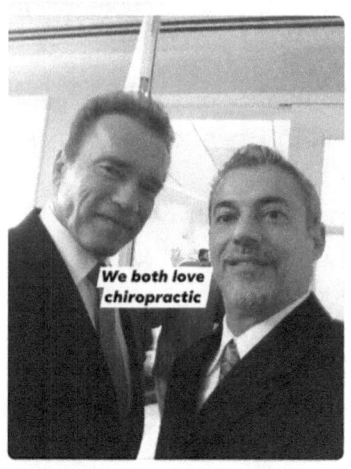

We both love chiropractic

Arnold, a great chiropractic promotor.

When we start to workout on a daily basis and develop our routines, after 21 days it is said that our routines become habit. The accumulation of good habits over long periods of time create a compound effect in our life in regards to obtaining better physical fitness therefore, with time, it really starts to show itself after 18 months. Imagine that you put forth just .01 percent more effort each day toward your fitness goals. Not 10 percent not 1 percent but just a tenth of 1 percent = .01 percent.

That is really a small extra effort. However if you are doing that every day of the month, after 30 days you will probably not even notice the 3 percent change in your fitness levels and/or changed reflection in the mirror or numbers on a scale. After 12 months or 365 days, you now have obtained a 36.5 percent change in fitness overall with that small .01 percent accumulated over the year. That is a noticeable number! 1/3rd better shape only after 1 year with a small effort, what if you did 10 percent versus .01 percent, get it? Now is the time to start moving more than anything. Create your why and go for it. Get off the couch, move it or lose it, your health depends on it.

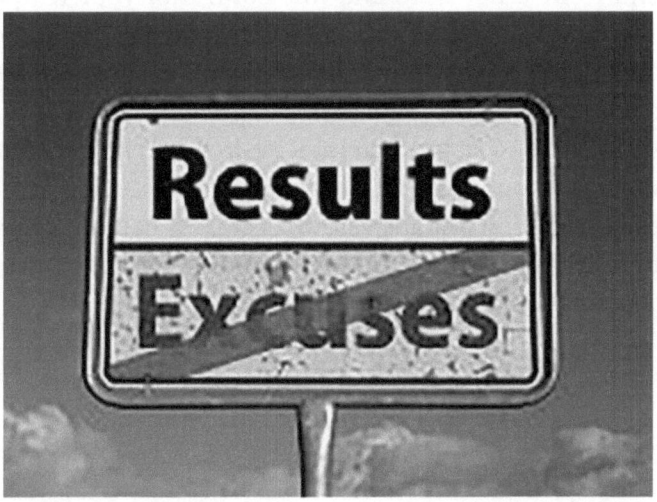

Exercise is not just for you but for the whole family too:

In a Swedish study, data was collected from over 1 million men. Those who performed regular cardio-fitness exercise scored higher in an IQ test.

Also 18 adults who led a sedentary lifestyle scored higher on multi-tasking, goal management, event planning, task switching, able to concentrate longer, just to name a few, after exercise was introduced into their life style on before and after test analysis. In other words physically fit individuals have an increased ability to focus better than those who live a sedentary lifestyle, these results were from a 2004 study.

In 2009, results of a study on aerobic activity were favorable toward showing the participants to have an increase in mental speed, attention, and cognitive flexibility.

In 2013, in the British Journal of Sports Medicine, a study was conducted to show that exercise was favorable to increase your willpower, self-control, problem solving and memory recall; in age groups 35 and younger.

In a 2 month study with a group that regularly showed emotional outburst of anger and frustration, after exercise was introduced into their lifestyle all participants showed an increased ability to control anger and had feelings on better mood and happier emotions. So if you tend to be a hot head and lose control of your temper often while blowing up at people, start exercising and get jogging immediately. This will not only be good for the people around you and those who you love but for your own personal growth too.

A study in 2014 showed an increase in short term memory after 30 moderate workout sessions. This can help the student achieve better grades for recalling test answers on exams. When biking was done for 35 minutes, long term memory was also improved even when after 4 hours passed from a learned topic.

"When exercising please wear black,
because this is a funeral for your fat."
(Jeff Trigo, DC)

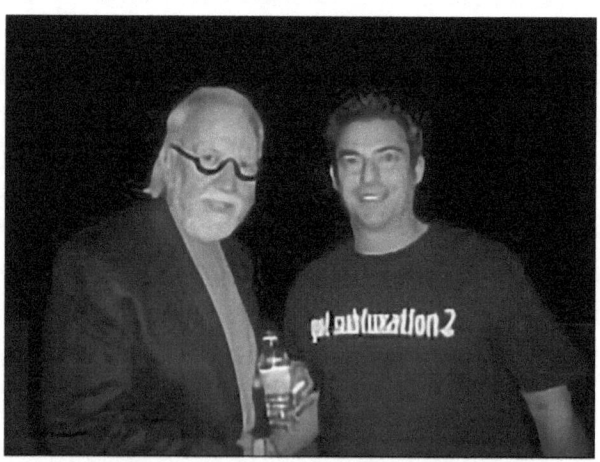

Dr. Jim Sigafoos, D.C. with Dr. Jeff Trigo, D.C.

I want you to write yourself a love letter. In the contents of this letter I want you to write a sincere apology for your lack of fitness discipline and promise yourself to get that body of yours into the best shape it has ever been in, no matter what age you are. What are you waiting for, go get that pen and paper.

Exercise is the way to get the most out of your brain, both mentally and physically. It will absolutely help combat disease, fight against depression, anxiety, stress, gives you a positive outlook on life while elevating your mood. You would love to be happier and healthier, all of us do, well this doesn't happen by chance, it takes good old fashion regular action to get your body in motion and once you've begun you're already half done. In other words, beginning is sometimes the hardest step, just begin, it will be a new habit in twenty-one days.

Most people don't know these benefits in regards to regular exercise:

During the International stroke conference of 2008, The American Stroke Association showed that healthy cardiovascular men and women who did regular moderate exercise had a 40 percent less chance of having a stroke.

In one of the longest studies of its kind, 35 years, Professor Brayne found that in 2000 men, regular exercise was the single most important contributing factor, amongst the healthy habits they acquired over their lifetime, in reducing and preventing dementia by a huge 60 percent. Also shown in the study was that inactivity can increase your chance of getting dementia by 82 percent. Also revealed was that if you only exercised once a week for 1 hour the risk of dementia was cut in half. I say do more than once a week. Three to five days a week is the minimum standard I would like to set for a healthier public with five to six days a week being the goal.

Other studies showed a change in healthier eating habits in those whom participated in regular exercise. This is a welcomed and awesome side effect. When one trains regularly, their consumption choices change to healthier choices due to the sweat equity and their greater desire to not sabotage their workout efforts thus creating a two-fold healthier you.

"The higher your energy level, the more efficient your body. The more efficient your body, the better you feel and the more you will use your talent to produce outstanding results." (Tony Robbins)

A study was performed on over 200 white collar workers to see if there were positive effects on employee output if they exercised before work or during the lunch break. Observed was increase in employee productivity, better moods, improvement in time management and increased employee tolerance toward co-workers. On the days that the people were inactive these observed benefits were not seen.

Another study from Bringham Young University observed different factors that contributed to lower productivity in the workplace in approx. Twenty thousand employees. Results showed that individuals whom only exercised occasionally or not at all were the ones that had decrease in productivity versus those employees who exercised on a regular basis.

"Take care of your body; it's the only place you have to live." (Jim Rohn)

Being a sedentary person can hurt you. In fact research is showing that being lazy is an absolute independent health risk and a study published by the Mayo Clinic Proceedings found that those who are physically active and fit are less likely to have adverse health effects from a sedentary lifestyle. So limit your couch and TV time, and/ or be active while watching TV. By doing sit ups, stretching on the floor, walking in place while high stepping, etc.

"I hated every minute of training, but I said don't quit. Suffer now and live the rest of your life as a champion." (Muhammad Ali)

A study conducted in 2014 showed that moderate to vigorous exercise programs showed to help with abstinence in drug addiction. Also observed was that people who exercise regularly had a lessen chance of drug use of any kind. Self-esteem was increased by exercise and the overall feeling of well-being was observed; which led to a lower incidence of drug use.

Studies also showed that in drug users, alcohol abusers and smokers, when exercise was introduced, the withdrawal symptoms were easier to overcome and cravings were greatly diminished.

**"Life is like riding a bicycle. To keep your balance,
you must keep moving."
(Albert Einstein)**

There are other benefits to exercise that involve improved learning. With exercise you acquire a sharper memory, improved learning skills, memory retention and an increased rate at which one learns. A 20 percent increase in speed in which one learns was seen in the groups in which exercise was implemented. This also led to improved academic performance and a higher chance of high school students enrolling in college. The largest results, 59 studies, came from those who did aerobic type of exercises. Body Mass Index (BMI) has been the standard of use in which one would assess ones physical fitness, however a low BMI measurement (low fat on the body), was not as good of a source in predicting ones fitness. The facts are that being physically fit (cardio-vascular via aerobic endurance) had better performance on test scores versus BMI.

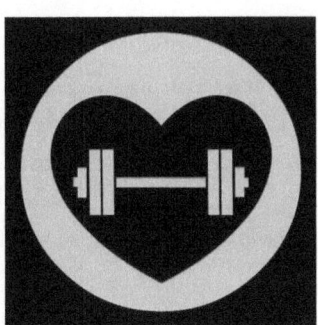

"If you always put limits on everything you do, physical or anything else. It will spread into your work and into your life. There are no limits. There are only plateaus, and you must not stay there, you must go beyond them." (Bruce Lee)

Key points to keep in mind is that nobody wants to exercise when they are in pain and that is why it is so important to take care of you spine. Regular adjustments will keep away spinal pain and inflammation thus propelling you to the gym with motivation and purpose. Move that body and live pain free. Pinched nerves will shut down the power of your shoulders, arms and legs thus inhibiting any great workout. VSC will cause a pounding headache, who wants to work out when they have a migraine? No one, therefore get adjusted and remove all excuses. Stay adjusted and enjoy an active lifestyle free of symptoms and reap the benefits that you read in this chapter. Never go longer than 2 weeks without an adjustment because subluxated spinal regions cause the disc to start drying up within that short period of time, and therefore injury is very probable. Develop your why, which is the purpose for getting in the best shape of your life, and use it as a motivating tool daily. Rip pictures out of magazines of the body you want and post it in various places. Set obtainable goals with time tables that are realistic and celebrate your achievements. And remember this important fact:

**"Rome wasn't built in a day but they worked
on it every single day." (Yuri Elkaim)**.

01 percent more effort daily will inch you steadily toward your goals and the only thing that can stop you is yourself. A last place finish is way better than did not finish which is way better than never started. Ready, Set, Go. Move that body, and dance like nobody is watching, celebrate that you have air in your lungs today and that you're very capable to move that body, and never stop!

**"It is a shame for a man to grow old without seeing the beauty
and strength of which his body is capable." (Socrates)**

Final words of encouragement: Keep a journal of your daily exercise. What muscle groups are being trained and how far did you run; how long did it take, etc. How many push-ups or pull-ups were you able to do? You can also track weight gain or loss. You can time your workouts and see how many repetitions you were able to accomplish in one minute. What was your BMI or blood pressure prior to starting your work-out commitment? What is the size of your pants prior to starting that long term physical training program? Logging this information will be a motivational tool to keep you engaged in physical fitness as you see these numbers start to show great improvements. Remember, I've said it before, it's not about the weight you lose, it's is all about the life you gain. Tap into the warrior within and ask your physician how you can safely get off any pills that may be hindering your wellness expression. Chose a natural safe and holistic approach to health instead.

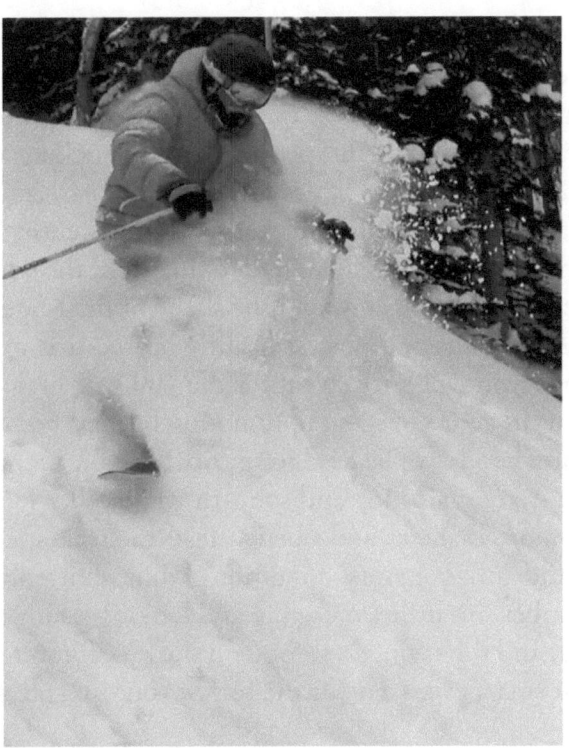

Vincent G. Ortega
Shredding Breckenridge since 1984

CHAPTER 9

Eat Well

You have heard this saying so many times, "you are what you eat." I'm beginning to think that there is so much truth to this statement. I have noticed that the people that are sucking down soda, and eating fried food, burgers, desserts and the sorts, smell and look different than those who consume real food consistently. People with clean pure real food diets have better looking skin, the whites of their eyes glow, have endless energy, and the shape of their figures are usually on the leaner side and possess healthy hearts. It is my hope that in this chapter you will learn to eat for the 100 year lifestyle, that the foods you put in your mouth are promoting life and not robbing you of your future. Foods can be used for growth, repair, strength, longevity, immune system boosting and so forth while other foods can clog arteries, promote diabetes and obesity, lead to strokes, contributing toward painful inflammatory conditions while shortening your life span. Remember this little tip, feeling and looking good is better than tasting good, and the saying "a second on the lips, forever on the hips; well then eat smart every day for the rest of your life, please.

How do you build up your bank account? By putting something in it every day. Your health account is no different. What I do today, I am wearing tomorrow. If I put inferior foods in my body today, it's going to be inferior tomorrow, it's that simple. (Jack LaLanne)

I want you to experience a change in what your body craves. Get addicted to healthy foods while learning that great taste exists in these healthy choices also. Keep in mind that it takes twenty-one days to create a new habit therefore we can apply this toward our food choices also. To see the compounded effect in our newly acquired healthier choices you continue to make you will need to continue this life style change, a.k.a. eating well habit, for at least 18 months. Then you'll be able to really notice a different you. Keep going, in three years its effects are very evident, in 10 years you are not the same person anymore, as all new cells that were reproduced, did so with great nutrition building blocks. In other words red blood cells last 120 days, well under great nutrition the reproduction of these cells are healthier. In a short amount of time, like a week, stomach lining is always being manufactured, our body continues to remodel bone cells and distribute it where it is needed while reabsorbing it as well. Under healthy nutrition this process of metabolism is under stronger and more efficient control. That is how you can experience a change in energy levels, skin tone, vibrancy, strength, radiance and longevity. It's a worthy task to learn what is good for the body and what is toxic. Wouldn't you want to know if a product you were eating was causing your illness, or feeding your cancer, or aiding in the spread of the disease? The Information you are about to learn can change lives. If one would just adjust their thinking and remember to stay adjusted, eat well and think well, the possibilities are endless.

Alkaline or Acidic Diet:
Alkaline foods fights against premature aging, cancer and disease while acidic foods supports disease, accelerated aging and cancer. It is wise to eat for health. I hope that you are learning many important factors that must be maintained to express wellness at optimum levels. Don't forget that besides alkaline foods, one must get adjusted. Chiropractic will maintain nerve supply and joint motion at 100 percent function which is vital for the expression of a wellness lifestyle. Exercise for charging our brain, the body's power plant to maintain full function and capacity while adding body tone, heart health and energy. Maintain an alkaline blood Ph. level for maximum long term

health benefits. This can be monitored via urine dip stick measurement of body Ph. Keep those levels alkaline and gain a disease fighting edge. I hope you are excited about what's ahead, because there are so many more gems in future chapters! If you are enjoying this book please tell others, every soul and every spine matters together we can change lives.

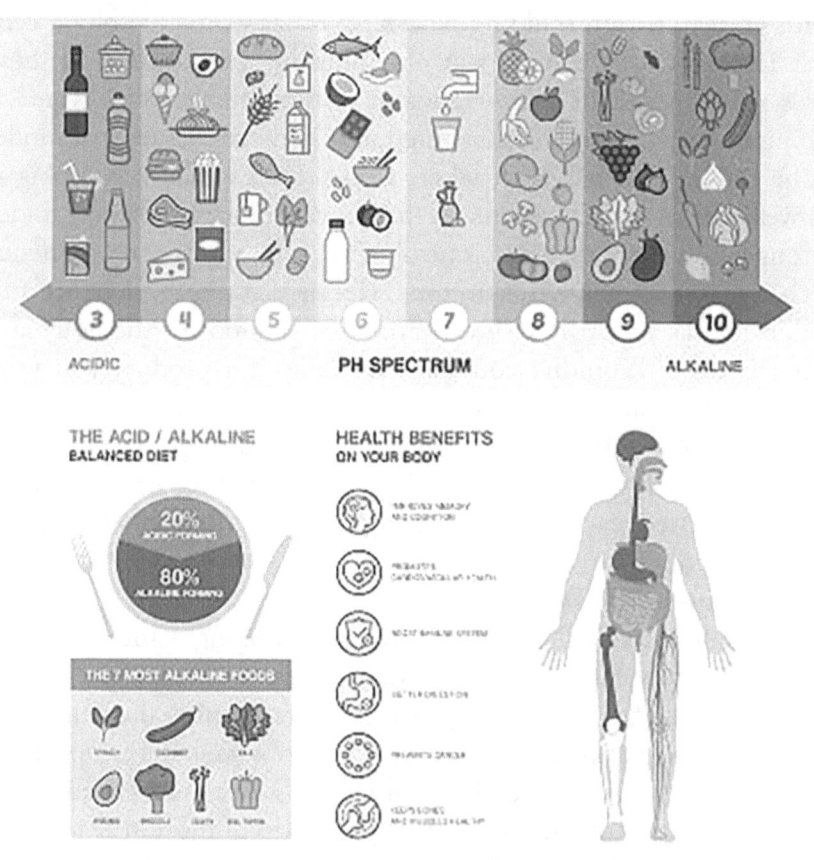

The Diet for the Diabetic: It's a difficult task to eat a well-balanced meal when you have diabetes because everything we consume will have the effect of either spiking or dropping blood sugar levels. What is most important is to make healthy choices while monitoring your portion size. A diet that is high in fiber has shown to help regulate blood sugar levels and aid in arterial health. Some of these high fiber foods include apples, artichokes, broccoli, Brussels sprouts, cauliflower, onions and seeds: chia, flax, pumpkin, sunflower, etc. To help regulate insulin more efficiently it is useful to eat some unripe digestive resistant carbs like bananas, mangos and papayas. Consumption of dark leafy greens have a benefit that are high in magnesium and potassium which have shown to be helpful in balancing blood sugar levels. Antioxidants help maintain healthy blood glucose levels and aloe vera can help prevent hyperglycemia. Cinnamon in large amounts has shown to be able to lower blood glucose levels naturally and ginger can lower you blood fasting glucose concentrations. Stevia is a natural sweetener and helps to regulate blood sugar levels. Stevia has also shown to help regulate insulin production and is considered a healthy sugar substitute. The diabetic must also eat a fair amount of healthy fats like avocados, salmon, sardines, nuts, olives, and grass fed meats, coconut oil and eggs. Exercise plays an important role in controlling diabetes and eliminating the amount of grains, sugars, bread, pasta, rice, sodas and juice you consume is crucial. Balance your gut with healthy fermented drinks with probiotics and supplement with antioxidants daily. Many diabetics have been able to reverse this condition and get off insulin by natural applied life style changes.

"Sugar is eight times addictive as cocaine." (Mark Hyman, MD)

Prayer doesn't change God, it increases our insight, perception, expands consciousness and totally transforms our inner persona. (Jeff Trigo, D.C.)

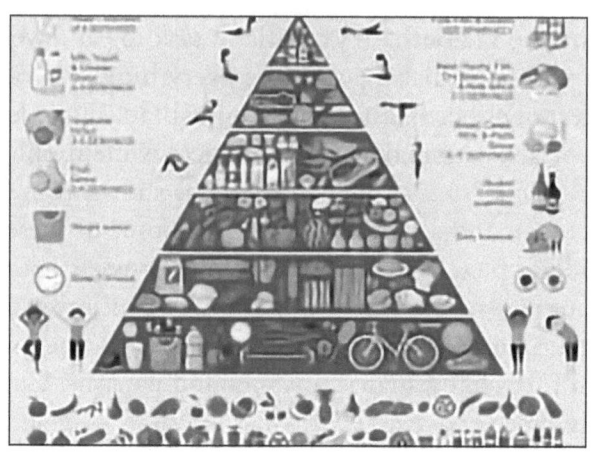

A Food Pyramid That Makes Sense:

The food pyramid that the USDA came up with years ago made people overweight. Eating that many servings of breads and grains per day will increase the mass of anyone. In a Mediterranean type of food pyramid, there is an abundance of the foods found naturally on the planet. Baked goods are absent in the Mediterranean type of diet thus the weight stays off. Bread will do one thing for sure if you consume it on a regular basis; build adipose tissue to your mass. The body stores fat in case of starvation. You see consumption of healthy fats will not make you gain weight, sugars do. Complex carbohydrates, a.k.a. sugars are the fat making culprit. Breads are this type of carbs, as is pastas, other baked goods, fudge, ice cream, cake, cookies, chips, etc. Table sugar, argh, an evil friend of diabetes and obesity, avoid it like the plague.

To try and make this information stick, let me give you this little bit of news: Sugars have a twelve-hour half-life when compared to fats which only have a 3 minute half-life. So for simple math during this example, let's say you ate 100 sugar calories. In 12 hours, balance is 50 cal. Add 12 more hours, balance 25 cal. Twelve hours more the balance is 12.5cal., twelve hours more the balance 6.25cal... Do you see that we will easily reach 5 days with trace amounts left to go! That is a lot of work for you pancreas to do, making all that insulin, no wonder type 2 diabetic patients start making new cells without insulin receptors, this is called the process of "down regulation." Fats = a three-minute half-life. Easy math, burnt off and processed by energy in the same day, no storage or insulin needed, just keep the fats healthy fats.

Eating Fat Will Not Make You Fat: Cut down on the complex carbohydrates (bread, pasta, rice, sugar, baked goods, ice cream, etc.) and increase your HDL fats (fish, olives, avocados, nuts) and proteins. As you just learned fat metabolizes relatively quickly, burns readily to energy for the body and they will help the integrity of the arterial wall. Cholesterol (found in animal products only) helps the cellular membranes. Your body makes more cholesterol than you can eat. My grandma lived to be 102 and she ate 2 eggs every morning. The body is brilliantly designed so when there are dangerous oils in your body wreaking havoc on the arteries, cholesterol (LDL) have shown to repair inner linings from damages sustained over long term exposure to these harmful entities. Change your oil cooking habits, stay adjusted, work out and know you are on the road to change for the better if you keep on it. Anti-oxidants will help arterial health I suggest Grape Seed Extract at 95 percent proanthocyanidins needed to be consumed at high doses say 50–100Mg per 50 lbs. This will return stretch to the artery vessels! Resveratrol is also an anti-aging powerful anti-oxidant. This helps reduce emboli and stroke; these anti-oxidants have also shown to reverse diabetic retinopathies, a condition in which causes loss of vision in diabetic patients.

The origin of our calories:

> Carbohydrates: 1 gram = 4 calories
> Proteins: 1 gram = 4 calories
> Fat: 1 gram = 9 calories
> Alcohol: 1 gram = 7 calories

This may be help full when calculating that the average 170 lb. man needs 2700 calories a day to maintain his weight. Increased activity means increase in calories needed and vice versa; 3,500 calories burned during exercise = 1 pound of weight loss.

Mind your Oils and Fats:

Type of Oil	Smoke point		Beneficial Information
Flaxseed oil	107C	225F	1:4 Omega 6–3 ratio
Safflower oil	107C	225F	133:1 Omega 6–3 ratio
Soy oil	160C	320F	GMO
Walnut oil	160C	320F	5:1
Hempseed oil	165C	330F	3:1
Butter	177C	350F	9:1 saturated fat
Coconut oil	177C	350F	86 percent Healthy saturated
Vegetable shortening	182C	360F	Unhealthy saturated and Trans fats
Lard	182C	370F	11:1 high in saturated fats
Macadamia nut oil	199C	390F	1:1 80 percent monosaturated Omega 9
Canola oil	204C	400F	3:1 GMO Mostly Polyunsaturated
Sesame seed oil	210C	410F	42:1
Extra virgin olive oil	216C	420F	13:1 74 percent Monosaturated Omega 9
Grapeseed oil	216C	420F	676:1
Almond oil	216C	420F	Omega 6 only
Hazelnut oil	221C	430F	75 percent Monosaturated, Omega 9
Peanut oil	227C	440F	32:1
Sunflower oil	227C	440F	40:1 Omega 6–3 ratio
Avocado oil	271C	520F	12:1 70 percent Mono, Vitamin E

Oil Summary: Use extra virgin olive oil for salads of when adding flavor to already cooked foods, however don't cook with it due to its lower smoke temperatures. Always look for organic cold pressed unrefined oils. When cooking in the middle range temperatures coconut oil is best or virgin olive oil, grape seed oil and/or small amounts of butter. When high temperature cooking is being done, like chicken cutlets, searing meats, using woks to cook or fry, etc., use avocado oil due to its very high smoke temperatures.

> **"Medicine is not health care, Chiropractic with nutrition and exercise is health care, medicine is sickness care." (Jeff Trigo, DC)**

The Raw Diet: It is suggested that heating your foods destroys some of the beneficial fibers, enzymes and nutrients that vegetables are helpful in for the fight against chronic disease and inflammation. Studies show that these enzymes break down at 116F degrees or 47C. Food will be more flavorful if you eat them raw while becoming more beneficial for longevity and no cooking was needed so clean up is easy. Did you know raw foods are cheaper to buy and quicker to eat while promoting health at the same time. I like to dip my raw veggies in hummus.

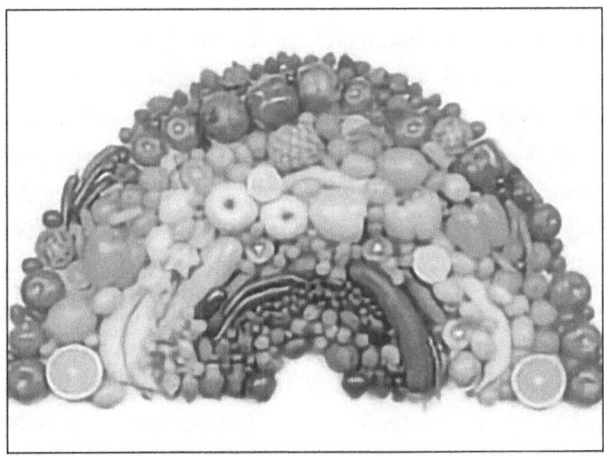

Eat the Rainbow:

It is so pleasing to the eye and healthy for the body to eat an abundance of different colors on a serving plate. Mix it up and have fun. Include beets, carrots, tomatoes and leafy greens with your main entre.

Morning breakfast: Range free eggs are always a great choice, a.k.a. pasteurized. Italian coffee that's not burnt or bitter. Add almond milk if desired. A favorite around the world is also green tea. Berries, fruits, bananas, persimmons, apples, pears, grapes, seasonal ripe fruits, etc., are highly suggested. Yogurt and fruit combo, oatmeal with nuts and seeds are both healthy alternatives.

Noon lunch: Turkey wraps with greens, shredded cabbage and carrots, hummus, avocado, olive oil and balsamic vinegar. Tuna is great, don't forget the lemon also try to avoid the bread if you can. Add chopped pickles, onions, celery, even hard boiled eggs. Vegetable omelets with mushrooms and greens can be eaten anytime of the day. Enjoy plenty of salads with chicken or fish, avocados, olives, chick peas, cranberries, and seeds, etc. Eat kale with tabbouleh salads. You can munch on hummus with whole wheat pita. Lean meats and fish are always a good choice when your inner carnivore craves.

Evening dinner: Eat wild caught fish often. Serve a wonderful salad with mixed greens and avocados, a fan favorite, seeds, veggies, etc. You can put protein and colors in salads too. Try an assorted greens mix with added: chopped beets and shredded carrots, dried cranberries, sesame seeds, pecans, cherry tomatoes, chopped cucumber (I like it half peeled). I suggest using an old Italian family favorite of a virgin robust olive oil mixed with balsamic vinegar 1/3 less versus oil mix, with some added chopped garlic for that extra kick. Make the dressing first, chop the garlic clove(s), put them into a container, add oil and vinegar, add a dash of Himalayan pink salt and fresh ground pepper and let it sit while you then prepare the salad. Dressing will absorb the garlic and mature in taste. Next prepare the salad ingredients, meanwhile your dressing is fermenting or curing and/or reacting with the garlic clove and awaiting your taste buds. It's a real treat, flavors from Italy, made in your own kitchen. Other salad additives I enjoy depending on what is available in the kitchen are: Kidney beans, chick peas, peas, artichoke hearts, fish or chicken, etc. Other healthy dinner options for the main dish includes beans and legumes, lean grass fed meats, baked vegetables, etc.

Eat this often: Cage free chicken eggs, greens, natural grass fed lean meats like beef, lamb, bison, elk, deer, etc. Wild caught fish. Eating mushrooms, avocados, and sprouts will also aid in better health. Keep a regular assortment of fruits and raw vegetables at the ready. Fermented foods, probiotics, and raw butter are helpful for normal digestion. Eat nuts and seeds. Foods high in antioxidants need to be on the top of the daily intake goals. Remember to consider the source.

Portion size: Be aware of serving amounts stated on labels. If the label reads serving size 8oz and it's a 16oz beverage, then whatever the calorie count is, keep in mind that this is for one serving, 8oz, so double it if the whole beverage is consumed. A meat portion is usually the size of your palm; 5–6 oz. It is also smart to use smaller plate sizes with meals, this allows for less food to be piled on if you are trying to lose weight. If you are in training then many calories are being burnt off during the strenuous training sessions, therefore calorie counting is not so important, just keep it real and wholesome foods found naturally in nature.

Protein Power: When we break down protein in our body we are left with amino acids, these are the building blocks to protein. Every cell in your body has protein in it as a component. We use protein to repair and build tissues, make enzymes, hormones and other important chemicals that our body needs for proper function. Protein is needed to form blood, bones, muscles, cartilage, soft tissues, organs and skin. Protein will also boost immune system function and help with the burning of fat with an added benefit of lowering your risk for diabetes. The recommended daily allowance for protein is 0.8

grams per kilogram of body weight or .36 grams per pound; 56–61 grams are needed for the average 170 lb. man, and 46–51 grams for the average size female. However in the USA where people weight more than in other places of the world the average size man is 195.5 lbs. while the woman is 166.2 lbs. Therefore a bit more protein may be necessary.

Healthy Sweet Choices: It is very common for people to have a sugar craving. This sweet desire is hard to quit because the urge is so strong and pleasurable for our taste buds. Unfortunately this can lead to increase in acidic environment within your body, while creating out of control binge eating. This habit is even worse if it's a late night binge when you're getting ready to retire for the evening and become sedentary while sleeping with all those extra calories in your system. Sugar turns into fat and needs insulin to get stored, so remember that always. It takes a lot of exercise to burn it off. I have found some really delicious alternative sweet treats that are natural and great tasting. The first food that comes to mind is ripe sweet fruit like berries, strawberries, mangos, grapes, watermelon, pears, apples, etc. These fruits are packed with nutrients and fibers. They are low in sugar and due to the high fiber content they will serve as a benefit to the artery cleaning process. Other sweet treats I enjoy are dates and figs. Dates and prunes are high in nutrients and are a great source of fiber, potassium, iron, and other beneficial plant compounds. One serving size is approximately three dates so don't eat too many, they are sweet and should satisfy any sweet tooth craving. Adding 3 dates to your yogurt and some chia or flax seeds are also healthy alternatives. The yogurt is rich in protein and calcium while the chia seed bring omega 3's fatty acids into the diet while absorbing water in the gut and giving you a feeling of being fuller longer. Sweet potatoes are filling, loaded with vitamin A, C and potassium. Fermented foods help regulate and balance gut bacteria while lowering the craving for sugars. Last but not least a small square of 70 percent or higher dark chocolate. This sweet snack has proven beneficial in its anti-inflammatory effects and anti-aging because it's an antioxidant, all beneficial to your health.

"You don't have to cook fancy or complicated masterpieces— just good food from fresh ingredients." (Julia Child)

When shopping in the grocery stores, stay in the outer areas because in the aisles you will only find bags, boxes, cans, and frozen foods, etc., and they are loaded with preservatives, ingredients we can't pronounce and are designed to have a long shelf life, but not offer you a long human life in any way! Keep the ingredients to five or less. Shop more often so you can have fresh produce and vegetables always available in the home. Buy different colors because different fruits and vegetables bring various different nutrients, vitamins and fibers; much needed elements that maximize your health and wellness potential. Try foods from other cultures (Asian, Persian, European markets) and buy a cook book if needed. There are always local stores that carry a different variety of fruits and vegetables.

"Your diet is a bank account. Good food choices are good investments." (Bethenny Frankel)

Proper Food Combinations: I like to maximize the benefits of eating foods that have similar digestive times in our stomach. In other words when food enters our stomach after being chewed, stomach acids go to work to further break them down into smaller more absorbable particles. Some foods break down fast and want to leave the stomach and enter the digestive track but cannot when combined with other foods that take several hours to break down. The food that gets broken down fast is stuck in the stomach fermenting while the foods that take longer to break down are still being digested. This can cause indigestion, bloating, and other GI symptoms. I recommend the following laws for food combining during meal planning:

1. Eat your proteins without the consumption of starches. Proteins are you meats; fish, chicken, beef lamb, etc. Starches are your breads, pastas, rice, potatoes, baked goods, noodles, grains, flour, tortillas, and corn. Starch takes 2 hours to break down and proteins take 3 hours. This means that

you can have proteins but must wait 3 hours before eating starches and if you are eating starches first you should wait 2 hours before the consumption of proteins.

2. Avoid eating fruits and vegetables at the same time. Fruits are simple sugars that break down faster versus starches that are complex sugars and take more time in the digestive track. Fruits can be eaten 30–60 minutes before a meal and never, I repeat never, eat dessert after a meal. Desserts tend to rot in the stomach; a sure way to get indigestion and heartburn. There is an exception to this rule and that is vegetables that have seeds in them act like fruits and can be eaten with other vegetables, they are called fruit vegetables: avocados, bell peppers, cucumbers, eggplant, squash, tomatoes, and zucchini.

3. Water melon should be consumed all by itself as well as other melons because of their fast digestive times and not breaking down well with other foods.

"Eat SOUL Food: Seasonal, Organic, Unprocessed, and Local." (Jessica Bradley)

www.rootedpantry.com

Healthy Carbohydrates: Carbohydrates can be divided into 3 categories: Monosaccharides, Disaccharides, and Polysaccharides. To better understand the different types of sugar chains available it would make sense to create comparative examples with other objects for better understanding. Consider this: Steel cables holding 2 sugars together versus bamboo links versus a straw like connection. The steel cables are complex sugars, a.k.a. polysaccharides meaning many sugar molecules stuck together. These are starches, glycogen, cellulose and chitin; Harder to break down and usually stored off as fat cells. The bamboo links are disaccharides meaning two sugars stuck together; still hard to break down but a bit easier than the steel cables. These carbohydrates include table sugar, milk sugar and malt sugar. Any sugar that is a long or medium chain sugar like the poly and di sugars must first be broken down into their singular form and therefore digestion takes longer and usually involves the need for insulin. Monosaccharides are a single sugar carbohydrate, like that of the straw connection which is easy to pull apart, and can be directly dissolved and put into the blood stream.

A mono or simple sugar is found in fruit, honey and syrup. Too much sugar causes levels in the blood to spike putting the person in danger of insulin resistance that can be developed with high sugar intake over time. Simple sugars found naturally on the planet like fruit, etc., have an easy absorbable simple sugar called fructose in them and you get added vitamins and minerals with natural water content that is healthy for the body giving you the feeling of staying full longer versus the donut type of sugar which spikes insulin, adds fat and clogs arteries, etc.

"Fast food is popular because it is convenient, it's cheap, and it taste good. But the real cost of eating fast food never appears on the menu." (Eric Schlosser)

No matter how horrible your health is today the key to overcoming this is not about changing your circumstances or applying excuses. The way to overcome any health failures you are dealing with is by changing yourself. That takes a process and a steadfast readiness to become teachable. A true desire for change; if you are willing to do that and start applying more and more wellness habits to your everyday mundane tasks, then you have already changed directions toward that future wellness destination. A future that is very obtainable with small changes compounded daily over time.

How to Calculate the Basal Metabolic Rate (BMR): This is in reference to the number of calories needed per day to stay exactly the same weight. This number will include day to day activity, exercise exertion levels expended and calories needed to keep warm and metabolize while sleeping, 3 parts to this equation.

Take your weight and divide it by 2.2 to convert it to kilograms. Example 170lbs divided by 2.2 = 77.73KG this represents calories needed each hour so times it by 24 = 1865.52 to obtain our first number.

Add 10 percent for thermal effects of food (burning calories while you sleep, digesting, immune system function, keeping warm, etc.) 1865.52 + 186.5 = 2052.02 our second number.

Now comes the tricky part! How active are you? Choose from the following:

1. Couch potato = 10 percent
2. Desk job and gym 3 times a week = 30 percent
3. Active job and gym 5 days a week = 50 percent
4. Construction worker with heavy lifting all day and gym 6 days a week = 100 percent

Let's say you choose number 2 at 30 percent. Take your previous number of 2052.02 and add 30 percent to it. 30 percent = 615.61 + 2052.02 = 2667.63 calories a day to maintain your current weight. If you want to gain weight eat more healthy calories if you want to lose weight eat fewer calories and bump up activities of daily living and increase your exercise regimen.

Another measurement that's popular and amongst the many various methods of determining ones fitness is body fat percent, or Body Mass Index (BMI). Fat gets stored in various places on the body and these measurements, with age taken into account, will give you a range that will inform you if you are at risk for heart disease. Remember increase in weight means that the body must build many more miles of capillary veins to deposit and/or reabsorb this new adipose tissue. It's been said that each pound of fat your body mass takes on, another mile of pipes must be laid down. So now you need a bigger heart pump, the heart muscle grows (cardiomegaly). Strike 1. Bad eating habits clog the arteries and make the main artery that supplies blood to the heart, the coronary artery, smaller in diameter. Now remember the heart muscle is bigger now and needs more O2, but in fact its vessel diameter is smaller via clogging of the inner pipe, Strike 2. Mix with a bit of stress, which makes the blood thicker, viscosity increases, making it harder to pump, strike 3.

Add cigarette smoking, which causes vaso constriction (smaller lumen/hole size) and there is strike 4. You only get 3 strikes and you're out so I guess you're hitting foul balls and are possibly a walking time bomb. Take personal accountability and change. Many people love you and will be sad if you died young. Develop a very big "why" and go for it, love the only human body you will ever get.

Below are the acceptable levels and unacceptable levels of BMI:

2 Charts to interpret results: I like the later
one, more accurate assessment!

1. Women: Low Healthy Overweight Obese

20–40 years:	≤21%	21–33%	33–39%	≥39%
41–60 years:	≤23%	23–35%	35–40%	≥40%
61–79 years:	≤24%	24–36%	36–42%	≥42%

Men: Low Healthy Overweight Obese

20–40 years:	≤8%	8–19%	19–25%	≥25%
41–60 years:	≤11%	11–22%	22–27%	≥27%
61–79 years:	≤13%	13–25%	25–30%	≥30%

2. I believe this is a more accurate chart:

Low Body Fat	Ultra-Lean-Lean	Moderately Lean	Excessive Fat	Obese
≤14%	15%–21%	22%–30%	31%–40%	≥41%

How to measure percent of body fat:

Take an average measurement of your weight over the course of several days, you will find that on a very accurate scale that measure

1/10th of pounds, that weight varies from day to day. Calculate your body mass index using this conversion: Weight divided by height in inches squared times 703.

Example 1. 170 pound 54 year old man who is 5'9'

Pounds ÷ by inches squared or 69"X2.

170 ÷ (69 ÷ 2) or 170 ÷ 69 ÷ 69 = 0.03570678 X 703 = 25.10 percent

25.10 percent body fat on a 54 year old man = Overweight chart 1, Mod-Lean chart 2.

Example number 2. A 22 year old woman who is 5'2" in height or 62 inches, and weighs in at 130 lbs. 130 ÷ 62 ÷ 62 = 0.03381894 X 703 = 23.77 percent

23.77 percent body fat on a 23 year old female = Healthy chart 1, Mod. Lean chart 2.

When considering weight loss tactics, consider this, 3500 calories burned is one pound weight loss. A bit of daily exercise can easily burn 250 calories, while eating 250 less (approx. 2 slices of bread) per day would be a pound a week loss. 250 + 250 = 500 X 7 days a week = 3500 calories, or 1 pound a week, 52 pounds a year. The compound effect in action once again.

"Eat like your life depends upon it." (Jeff Trigo, DC)

When to buy organic: In today's agriculture methods, genetic modified organism (GMO) seems to save companies money while heaping poisonous pesticides upon their products then selling them to the unsuspecting public thus creating a whole new stream of diseases that seem to be linked to an increase of illness and loss of life expectancy. In the supermarket there are so many choices, organic costs more and should I buy that brand versus nonorganic and save a bit? Well let me make it simple for you, below is a list of the Dirty 13 items that should always be purchased as organic and the clean 14 than can be bought inorganic: March 2019

Dirty 13: Buy Organic
1. Strawberries
2. Spinach
3. Kale
4. Nectarines
5. Apples
6. Grapes
7. Peaches
8. Cherries
9. Pears
10. Tomatoes
11. Celery
12. Potatoes
13. Sweet Corn (GMO)

Clean 14: Buy non-organic
1. Avocado
2. Pineapple
3. Sweet Peas
4. Onions
5. Papaya
6. Eggplant
7. Asparagus
8. Kiwi
9. Cabbage
10. Cauliflower
11. Cantaloupe
12. Broccoli
13. Mushrooms
14. Honeydew

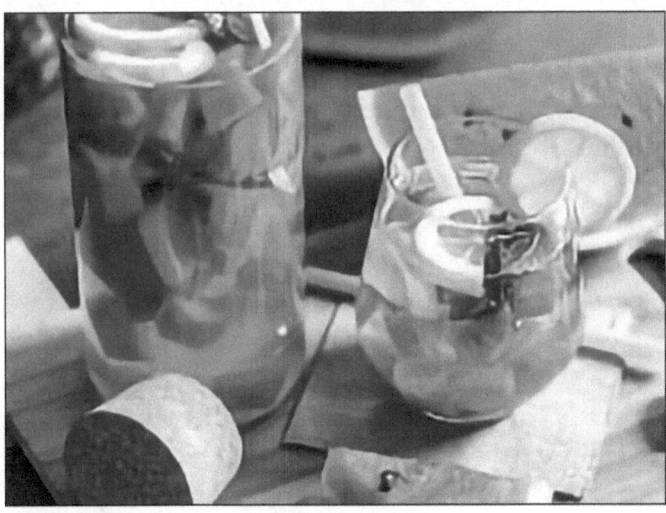

Apricot seeds contain vitamin B17 which have anti-cancer benefits as well as antioxidant properties.

CHAPTER 10

Think Well

We must learn to take every thought captive that enters our mind and filter it as being useful information or junk. There is so much trash that can bombard our daily thoughts and try to rob us of our daily joys. This is unacceptable! Rebuke the useless noise/distortion/feedback, and allow in only the thoughts that are in alignment with our integrity, goals and lifestyles that we are trying to attract to ourselves. Shut off gossip, run from that daily negative news report about death, violence and destruction. Where you focus your mind is what holds you captive. The real challenge is to think positive in a negative world. Inspire to seek stories that move you into action toward a greater good than self. Seek after knowledge as the greatest treasure on earth. To live well one must possess mental health.

"Whatever is true, whatever is honorable, whatever is right, whatever is pure, whatever is lovely, whatever is of good repute, if there is any excellence and if anything worthy of praise, let your mind dwell on these things." (Philippians 4:8)

"I say then: Walk in the Spirit, and you shall not fulfill the lust of the flesh." (Galatians 5:6)

The dog that wins the fight is the one you feed; so feed the Spirit daily.

"The grass is greener where you water it." (Pastor Chris Danell) www.ChurchOfNaples.org

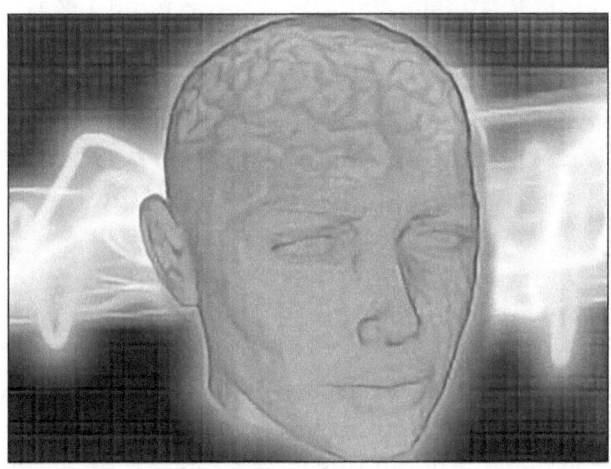

All things are possible with an increased serving of wisdom, just like King Solomon. In the Bible, 2 Chronicles 1:7–12, A worthy passage to read, Solomon seeks after wisdom to be a good king and not wealth or long life, etc., and because of this selfless act God gave him everything. If your heart is in the right place your thoughts will follow and dwell in that place also. Absolute mental health is being grounded in the Word, following His commands, and trusting in Him who loves you and wants to have a personal relationship with you. Be grounded in the Word.

Life is a journey and we must learn to enjoy the process not just the destination. Every day we must deliberately take the necessary steps to write down and/or review our goals, then embrace those actions needed to achieve your desired results. Learn daily, grow in knowledge daily and make the effort to become a better version of you today. The secret of your future is hidden in the daily routines and habits we create today. The lifestyles of the super-rich and wealthy differ greatly from that of a homeless person, however, wealth doesn't dictate any increase in joy and contentment. You can't buy your way into Heaven!

I know miserable rich people and awesome happy full of joy poor people. What's the difference? It's the heart and soul of the person that distinguish them apart. A healthy mind needs to be cultivated, and joyful folks seem to have a regular expression of faith while having a servant's heart toward others.

"Life is not just the passing of time. Life is the collection of experiences and their intensity," (Jim Rohn)

The type of work we do is not as important as the attitude we express while doing this work. We should be approaching every endeavor with the attitude as if we were working directly for God Himself. This attitude of excellence will get addicting while demonstrating an example to others as to the type of mettle we are made of. The apostle Paul wrote about this nearly 2000 years ago and it is still awesome advice today.

"Everything you do in life, I don't care, the good or bad— don't blame God, don't blame the devil, don't blame me, blame you. You control everything! The thoughts you think, the words you utter, the foods you eat, the exercise you do. Everything is controlled by you." (Jack LaLanne)

You heard it said that today is a gift, that is why it is called the "present." Tomorrow is a "promissory note" that day may never come because one day it will be your last. In regards to the past, its "gone", "over with" and only exists as a memory. You can't ever go there or ever find it again therefore learn from it, forgive at all cost and let it go! Forgiveness will do you more of a benefit than it can possibly ever do for someone else. It will take the elephant off your back and release so much negative emotions that slow you down and hinder real progress within. Use failure as a lesson of what not to do. Stop holding any grudges, put away your story that definitely has been most likely misinterpreted. There are always more than 1 side of a story. People can witness the same event and come up with entirely different meanings thereof. We are a bunch of meaning making machines. This is causing mass confusion as meaningless negative conclusions are being assumed thus breeding grief and despair as it rips apart relationships one by one. Stop it, change this reckless thought pattern, you can do this at any moment. Rebuke the negativity, and start practicing forgiveness in a Godly manner. It's actually biblical to forgive:

And be kind to one another, tenderhearted, forgiving one another, even as God in Christ forgave you." (Ephesians 4:32)

If this was actually followed it would change the world and make it a safer and happier place to live. Be the change you want to see in the world.

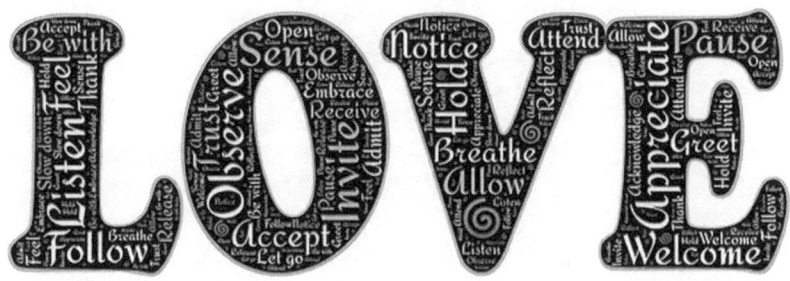

Communication is such a strong tool that can mend the biggest divides and allow for a greater reconnect in relationships. Imagine a gentle tone with a smile as an exhortation is being given. An exhortation is telling someone of a sin or wrongful act that they may be committing and doing it in a nonjudgmental loving way and don't forget the all-important loving smile. Another great communication tool includes plenty of "I" statements versus "you" statements. For example, "I feel that when you're always late it makes me feel like my time is not valuable and I feel disrespected", versus, you are always late, you don't respect my time, you will never change, etc. Keep your tone loving and try to repair the lost family relationships that Satan has managed to rip apart and start putting them on the mend. Who else will do this for you and improve the quality of your life? It is got to be the person in the mirror because no one else will do this for you. Results will naturally breed improved relationships and better mental stability in your life. It's nice when people enjoy being around you, always make your friends and family feel important to you, heck even strangers!

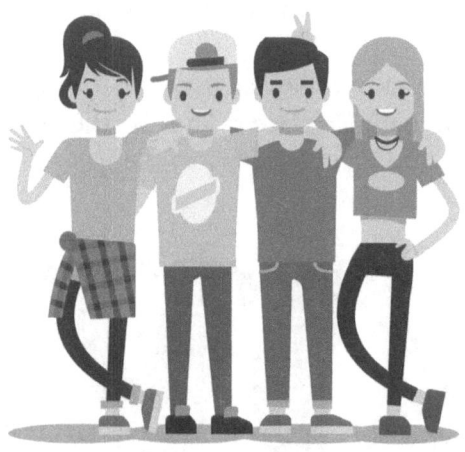

Unique Self: Did you know that there is just 1 you in the universe? Only one person with your exact DNA, only one with your face and personality. Only one with your life experiences and memories. You are a cherished individual! Angels and Demons are fighting over your very soul. With that kind of recognition in mind this should create a sense of worth to you the individual. You are a one of a kind gem that our great Creator desires to have a personal relationship with, therefore put away any thoughts of depression, anger and hate, etc. You are a trillionaire in Heaven if you believe in the forgiveness of sins that are gifted only by the blood that was poured out by Jesus on that Cross over 2000 years ago. Our life is but a vapor here today gone tomorrow. The life span of man is 120 years and then it's over forever. Most of us will never even see 90! If this is always kept fresh on our mind, then each day will be spent as if it were our last, giving

100 percent of our self to the day and creating a meaningful purpose driven life that serves a higher power other than self.

Celebrate each day as a new beginning. We have the opportunity to wake up each day forgiven, a totally clean slate, then we get out of bed! It is only the devil that wants you to think that you are not loved or that you're not good enough. This is not of God but from the liar from the beginning, Satan himself. Don't entertain these negative thoughts, throw them away to rebuke and praise the creator, God, instead. This daily practice will transform your thoughts into reality and create the updated version of you, the one with the great attitude of gratitude that will attract people like bees to honey. This will take a shift in where you focus your thoughts. Practice it today because you are an overcomer by faith, redeemed by the blood of the Lamb of God.

Goal Setting: Goals are like a compass, they keep your thoughts and eyes on a specific destination so that you always know where you are heading. With these goals, written down on paper, you will be able to fulfill your purpose in life and live your dreams. Each one of us has a purpose for which we were created. One of our greatest responsibilities is to identify that purpose, create a purpose driven life and experience great joy as we fulfill that purpose. A useful tool to help you identify what's your purpose is prayer. Pray without ceasing is what's best because it keeps you in the proper alignment with Gods will. Another useful tool for identifying that purpose is meaningful goal setting. I will give you the best goal setting tool I've have ever seen! If you take the time to do all of the steps necessary in writing these answers down on paper, you will have a better perspective on your purpose and what your heart really desires. There is no shortcut, or quick way to get through this, some of the questions may take time. Answer all of them and then you will be able to have a better understanding on the purpose for which you were created.

Keep in mind that simply achieving goals will not guarantee you any success or contentment. As you achieve your goals you will feel a sense of accomplishment with or without success. You see success is a journey not a destination. It's very important to have a dream, and goalsetting makes those dreams more of a reality and obtainable. I know that if you do this goalsetting exercise you will acquire a compass that can point you in a better direction; a direction with greater purpose with meaningful existence and increased satisfaction for life.

Please don't just read through this next goalsetting page. If you have to book mark it and come back to it later, that's ok. The only way I want you to read this next section is when you are prepared; sheets of paper and a pen at the ready. This exercise should define you. Reveal to you the things that really matter in life. Expose any circumstances that need closure, etc. Identify a path that needs to be taken to fulfill your purpose in life thus maximizing your JOY and eternal destiny.

> **"Goals. There's no telling what you can do when you get inspired by them. There's no telling what you can do when you believe in them. And there's no telling what will happen when you act upon them." (Jim Rohn)**

A dream or goal can be an amazing and incredible thing to have and achieve. It can motivate you and keep you going on the path when the going gets tough. It will provide a compass and direct you toward a destination that you may have never aspired toward or fathom. Just do me a favor, don't keep it as an ideal, you must take every action step necessary to make it become a reality. Continual and steady improvements will push you along the path of reaching your greatness potential. Everyday strive to be a little better than the previous day. This is the compound effect in motion propelling you along the journey of success and happiness. Smell the flowers along the way and sing praises to the living God.

> **"All Scripture is given by inspiration of God, and is profitable for doctrine, for reproof, for correction, for instruction in righteousness, that the man of God may be complete, thoroughly equipped for every good work." (2 Timothy 3:16–17)**

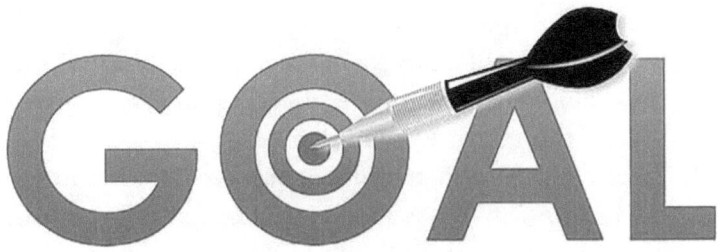

Goalsetting:

To start, go get a pen and blank booklet of papers.

1. Make a list of the 5 things you valued most: (what things would you fight for, what would you sacrifice the most for, etc.).
2. 3 Goals in 30 seconds-go.
3. If you had $ Ten Million dollars in the bank, what all would you do?
4. If you only had 6 more months to live, what would you do with that time?
5. What thing have you always wanted to do but fear has held you back?
6. What is it that you do that adds the most wonderful feelings and personal satisfaction in your life?
7. If you had 1 wish from a Genie, or what one great thing would you do or would you accomplish if you knew you couldn't fail?
8. Now make a list of 50 things:
   - What do you want to see, to do, to have, or to become?
   - Economical, material, personal, and professional goals.
   - Social goals, personal development, family goals, etc.
A) Rate each topic with a time frame attached to it: 1, 3, 5, or ten-year goal.
B) Rate the top 4 most important in each category.
C) Write a paragraph of "WHY"; the why of you wanting the goal is more important than the goal itself.

9. Write 10 Admonitions:

   Example: I enjoy loving my patients the way they love me, I enjoy dynamic health, and financial freedom is everything I thought it would be. Etc.

10. Take pictures next to your unachieved goals and visualize ownership with dates and a timeframe of achievement. The picture of you standing next to that RV you always wanted, that dream house, its cost etc. Put some Post-its up stating your goals in high visibility areas in the home such as a mirror, on the refrigerator etc. These are constant reminders to remain focused and press on.

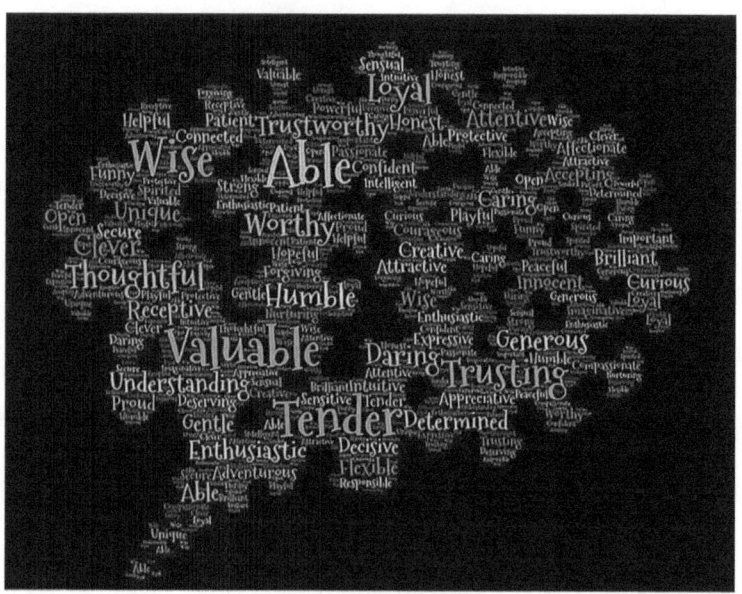

You can either try to be in control of every aspect of your life, micro-managing everything or you can simply let go and just trust. You can't be in control of your life and trust at the same time, it's a one or the other choice. I choose to trust a huge God capable of doing anything and everything! Feed the spirt and you will not fulfill the desires of the flesh which are contrary to one another. Having goals keep your inner compass pointing in a specific direction while prayer time puts you in alignment with Gods will for you and creates a personal relationship that lasts into eternity.

"Our goals can only be reached through a vehicle of a plan, in which we must fervently believe, and upon which we must vigorously act. There is no other route to success." (Pablo Picasso)

Hopefully by now you figured out that some of the questions get you to think deeply about what is most important in your life. Don't wait till you only have 6 months left to live to enjoy the satisfaction of righteous living and mended relationships. Do what's right and start benefiting from the life that God wants you to fulfill. Become the best version of you ever, and focus your energy on your goals. You heard of the 80/20 rule? The Pareto principle, a.k.a. 80/20 rule (the law of the vital few, or the principle of factor sparsity) states that, for many events, roughly 80 percent of the effects come from 20 percent of the cause. In other words, 20 percent of what you do will bring in the 80 percent success/income, etc. So focus on the 20 percent that is most effective and maximize that potential into a higher percent for better results. Do the main thing more often for best results and show JOY along the way. I like to say that joy stands for this: J = Jesus, O = Others, Y = You, and in that order will you find that you can become a person of greater influence thus affecting the lives of many around you.

"Setting goals is the first step in turning the invisible into the visible"
Tony Robbins

Set up weekly chiropractic appointments, and never go 14 days without an adjustment. Eat as healthy as possible; 99 out of 100 meals, and take your supplements; it will boost immune system optimization. Exercise 3–5 times a week, mix it up and have fun doing it. Brush, floss and water pik your teeth daily. Set big goals and go for it, life without fear! Tell someone how much you care about them today while celebrating that you're alive! Remember, God answers knee mail so get down and kneel often. Jesus will return again as promised, so look up to the sky with a smile, He is coming soon!

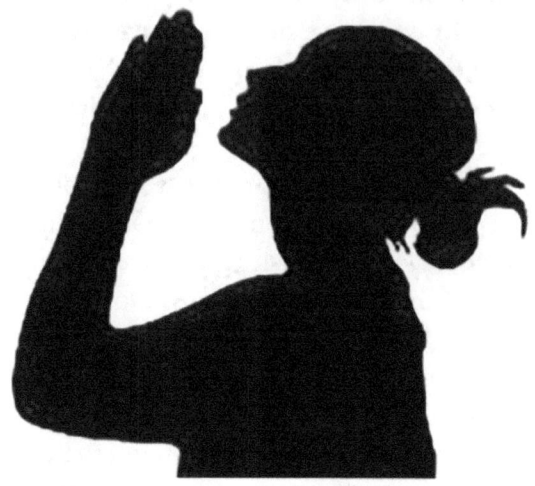

Prayer: The efficiency of our mental status is highly affected by those who have an active prayer life versus those who do not. Prayer can calm the storm and move the mountains. Prayer with great faith is like a muscle that can get stronger as you continue to engage in it. Pour into our Creator and He reveals Himself to you and you will feel His presents in a mighty way. It is said in the Holy Bible that without faith it is impossible to please God, therefore what is this faith? Simply put, faith is believing in something unseen. Belief that is not based on proof. With that said, it takes an act of faith to pray. The greatest gift is when God starts to answer those prayers and moves within your life as He refines you as you go through various trials, called life. This refining process will remove the impurities and make you more useful for His kingdom expansion purposes. Show me a worn out well read Bible and I'll bet its owner is the opposite of worn out and full of peace.

> **"And just as you want men to do to you,**
> **you also do to them likewise."**
> **Luke 6:31**

In order for prayer to work, there are some key ingredients that prayer must contain otherwise they won't travel higher than the ceiling as the voice sounds bounce off and travel no further! What are these key components that will take our prayers to the throne of the Most High and how can I maximize the efficiency of my prayer life? We can examine the way that Jesus prayed and find all the answers in our Bible. A common denominator with prayers is that it must be in the Nature of God, and it must glorify the Son. The Nature of God is love therefore it can't be a revengeful prayer, and should always bring glory to the Son, it's all about our Savior, not the self. The prayer must not be self-centered. How will this prayer move God and bring glory to His Son? So consider that when you pray to God the Father in Heaven, and always end your prayer like this, In Jesus name I pray, Amen. Remember the Trinity of God is bigger than our own comprehension. That's biblical so exercise some faith and trust in the biblical truths and its many prophecies that validate the scripture. Where 2 or more are gathered in prayer know that the God of the universe is with you in the midst. The squeaky wheel gets the oil, so don't give up, God loves you.

"That Christ may dwell in your heart through faith." (Ephesians 3:17)

Our awesome God exists in 3 different unique beings yet all in 1. The 3 in 1 mystery of the Holy Trinity is an act of faith. God the Father. God the Son, and God the Holy Spirit, three in one. Proof is found back in the first book of the Bible where it says:

"Let Us make man in Our image, according to Our likeness; let them have dominion over the fish of the sea, over the birds of the air, and over the cattle, over all the earth and over every creeping thing that creeps on the earth." (Genesis 1:26)

Jesus came to do the will of the Father and was obedient even unto death. He and the Father were of one accord, and even from the beginning all power of creation was giving to the Son to create the

Universe because it pleased the Father. Jesus, the master carpenter, left heaven to be born on earth to die for you and me.

The 8 S's:

1. Sinner: All have sinned and separated ourselves from our Holy God.
2. Salvation: We need a Savior to bridge the gap between Heaven and Earth.
3. Savior: His name is Jesus Christ, fulfilled more than 300 prophecies foretold before His birth. He was from the birth line of King David, the tribe of Levi, the Priestly line.
4. Sacrifice: He who knew no sin, our perfect sacrifice, the second covenant prophecy fulfilled that day on the cross. He paid a price that He did not owe, a debt that we could never pay. Obedient always to the Father's will, even death on a cross, thank you Jesus.
5. Sanctification: As we give ourselves to Jesus as our personal Lord and Savior (acknowledgment that we need a savior to get to heaven, confess our sins and be thankful for the forgiveness we are gifted by grace that we may boldly approach the Throne of God and receive mercy), He will pour into our life as we mature spiritually and become more Holy, the presents of the Holy Spirit in our fruitful lives, and living for the spirit not the flesh is the process of sanctification.
6. Set Free: No longer a slave to sin or death. Co-inheritor to the kingdom of God. Mansion in Heaven, where there is no more sorrow, death, or tears. Overcomers.
7. Saved: Assured 100 percent that when we take that last breath, we have citizenship in Heaven because of faith in the finished works of the cross of Jesus, my redeemer.
8. Service: As we grow in the faith, love, joy and develop a personal relationship with Christ, our Lord, we desire to give back out of the heart's natural yearning and start to serve a need at the church. This service can be in many forms.

Music ministry, if that's a talent, it can be in the children's ministry, clean up, soup kitchen, missionary field, etc. I have seen people watering the plants, picking up trash in the parking lots, directing traffic. It is always awesome to see God moving in the hearts of His people whom He dearly loves, what a blessing! Continue to embrace biblical truths, stay away from legalism because you will be labeled a hypocrite and let your words and actions match your integrity; Get involved today and stay authentic.

"For as the body without the spirit is dead, so faith without works is dead also." (James 2:26)

The Lord's Prayer: Talk about an example of how to pray. When the Lord prayed this prayer He did not intend this to be the only prayer we do like a robot and thus create a shallow predictable prayer life with no personality or intimate relationship with our Father in Heaven. Repetitious prayer is shallow and without heartfelt communication to our creator. It was a template and an example as Jesus said:

"After this manner therefore pray ye: Our father which art heaven, Hallowed be thy name. Your kingdom come. Thy will be done in earth as it is in heaven. Give us this day our daily bread. And forgive us our debts, as we forgive our debtors. And lead us not into temptation, but deliver us from evil: For thine is the kingdom, and the power, and the glory forever. Amen." (Matthew 6)

Worship: We were created to have a relationship with our creator. He demands worship and that becomes our privilege to sing praises to the King of kings and Lord of lords. When we sing the presence of the Holy Spirit makes Himself known in us by setting up His residents in our hearts. As He pours into us, we feel His presence and it's truly indescribable. The more you praise Him, our God, the more blessed you are and the worries of this world seem to just melt away. This is the glue to the relationship that makes it real, God in us, a saved human being, doing what we were created to do, worshiping Him. This personal relationship will be seen in you as you live a life that is heavenly minded not earthly grounded. Wake up singing praises to our Father. He enjoys hearing from us, in Jesus name, amen.

"God is a Spirit: and they that worship Him must worship Him in Spirit and in truth." (John 4:24)

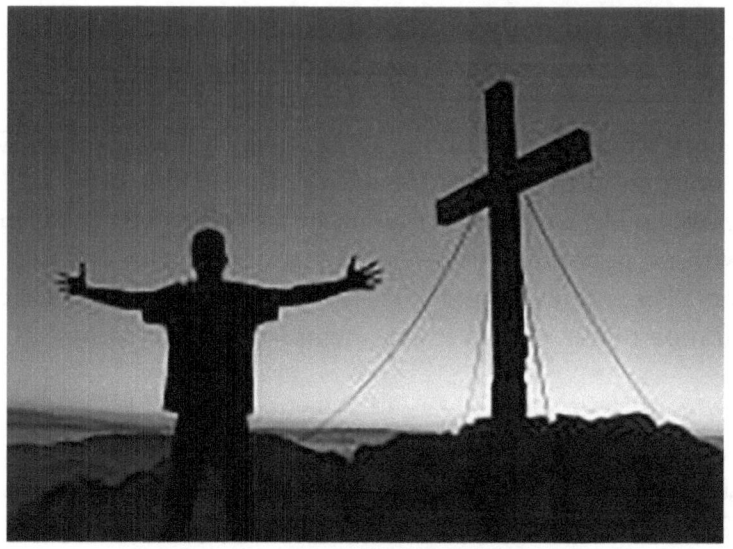

"Give unto the Lord the glory due unto His name; worship the Lord in the beauty of holiness." (Psalms 29:2)

Fellowship: Many great motivational speakers have said, "show me the 5 people that you spend most your time with and I will define who you are." Do you have friends that you respect? Are your friends looking out for your best interest? Do you all have the same moral compass? Do they care about your eternal destination and righteous living?

Do they possess the same ethical and moral values as you do; or maybe they have outstanding ethics and you need to get where they are? Fellowship is hanging out with likeminded Christ loving people, that are forgiven and desire to live a Holy life. Have you ever seen a stack of coals pile up on fire as the BBQ is getting ready to cook, then one of the coals falls away from the pack? The lone coal cools off and gets darker while the coals in the pack remain hot and glowing. This also happens in real life situations. People that leave the church start getting depressed, sin is easier, no one to hold them accountable, as they drift away to the dark side where the devil loves to accuse you of being worthless, useless and unlovable.

It's all lies! Get back into fellowship today. Surround yourself by people who love the Lord and are forgiven, and living a sanctified life.

"Give not what is holy to the dogs, nor cast your pearls before swine, lest they trample them under their feet and turn and tear you in pieces. Mathew 7:6

In other words if you put some pearls on a pig, and dress it up, it will still do what it does, lay around in the filth and mud. Same with the unsaved unethical friends you may be spending time with. They do not care that you are set apart and have overcome this world. They don't care that you have overcome death and sin by the power of forgiveness via Christ, and that the Holy Spirit lives inside you. They want you to join them in their sin and bring you down to their level. Misery loves company. Change your perspective regarding your friends, they need to be witnessed to and told that you are no longer that same person. Healthy and great minds think alike, surround yourself by people who are better than you to up your game. If they don't understand and respect your decision to live a righteous life and to become a better version of you then you're best off losing them, because they were never truly a friend to begin with. Choose quality over quantity, forget the 20 nickels; go find a few golden dollars instead.

Listen to encouraging music often, it feeds your soul and connects you to God through worship and praise.

Mental Health: The definition is as follows;

"…a state of well-being in which the individual realizes his or her own abilities, can cope with the normal stresses of life, can work productively and fruitfully, and is able to make a contribution to his or her community."
World Health Organization (WHO)

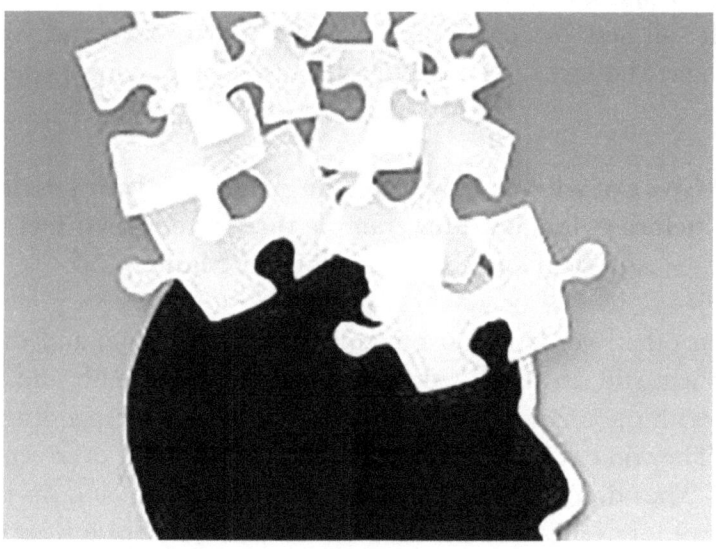

I truly believe that if you have God in your heart, you know where you are going when this world passes you by and you understand that you have been bought and paid for by the precious blood of Jesus—then you have a huge head start toward achieving a healthier mental status that allows you to function at a higher capacity. To know Christ is to know peace. And vice versa is true, no Christ, no peace. It's that simple. If you're depressed: pray, get adjusted, exercise and eat healthy. If this doesn't change the circumstance and your faith in God is still full of doubts, then get counseling. I am not a fan of psyche meds for mental issues, because their side effect are thoughts of suicide, but proper life style changes and Godly wisdom will do wonders for the thoughts of mind.

**"Ye are of God, little children, and have overcome
them: because greater is He that is in you, than
he that is in the world." (1 John 4:4)**

Remember we serve a very big and mighty God, never put Him in a box and limit His abilities to reveal Himself in a mighty way. He said to ask and you shall receive and He knows the status with all of His creations. He knows the number of hairs on your head before you were even conceived in the womb, all knowing, omnipresent, knows the past, present and the future; creation declares His Glory. Whatever your mental insecurity is, whatever is causing you mental anguish, or anxiety, leave it at the cross and do not pick it up again. He can take care of it for you. Pray without ceasing and with fasting when needed. When 2 or more gather in Christ name He is there amongst you so go find a prayer warrior and combine your prayers. Satan hates prayer groups because this hinders his evil ways.

The Whole Armor of God: No one ever said that life would be easy. In fact it is full of disappointments, hurt, pain and suffering, why? Because of sin that entered into the world long ago with Adam and Eve and it has been that way ever since. It's called a fallen state of man. This will change one day, upon death we will be absent the body and present with our Lord as we get to spend eternity in paradise, granted to those who overcome the sting of death via faith of the cross. This armor of God can help us to move off the bumpy roads of today's life that is filled with potholes, dead ends and cliffs by crossing over onto the smoother and blessed roads of life we travel. The Armor can equip us with the much needed protection as ongoing spiritual warfare between Angels and demons fight to win the souls of humans. Don't be caught naked when the fight comes to you, instead be dressed for battle:

"Finally, my brethren, be strong in the Lord and in the power of His might. Put on the whole armor of God that you may be able to stand against the wiles of the devil. For we do not wrestle against flesh and blood but against principalities, against powers, against the rulers of the darkness of this age, against spiritual host of wickedness in the heavenly places. Therefore take up the whole

armor of God that you may be able to withstand in the evil day, and having done all, to stand. Stand therefore, having girded your waist with truth, having put on the breastplate of righteousness, and having shod your feet with the preparation of the gospel of peace; above all, taking the shield of faith with which you will be able to quench all the fiery darts of the wicked one. And take the helmet of salvation, and the sword of the Spirt, which is the word of God; praying always with all prayer and supplication in the Spirit, being watchful to this end, with all perseverance and supplication for all in saints—and for me, that utterance may be given to me, that I may open my mouth boldly to make known the mystery of the gospel, for which I am an ambassador in chains; that in it I may speak boldly, as I ought to speak. Ephesians 6: 10–20

Daily Routine: Before bed time make a list of 20 things you need to accomplish the following day and on the back of the list add 3 things you need to be. Examples: more patient, happier, more sympathetic, practice being grateful. Etc. If you are making the list the same day then you are already behind, do it the day before. Cross off the task as you do them, get the big tasks out of the way early, and rewrite the list for the next day with any undone tasks on the top of the list as first priorities.

If you can master your day you will be able to master you week. If you're able to master your week then you can master your month. Those that are diligent to master their month can master their life! You are the architect, start building toward a better future today. To maximize mental health you must stay focused and busy moving toward your goals and dreams. The truth of a dream gives you strength to help others along the way while the fulfillment of a dream creates joy and purpose thus leading to mental contentment; happy at exactly where you're at right now. The journey ahead is awesome and it is filled with abundance, hope and happiness. Cultivate your dream and it will give you the promise of a better future, all you need is a dream and a plan to get started. Once begun, you're half done!

Church 101: We are sinful people serving a righteous God. Want to help someone—tell them the truth. Bibles says we are sinners and an enemy of God. If you die in your sin you're heading straight into hell. Give your life to Jesus. God hates our sin, so we need to be born again. Seek things above. Repentance is an actual change of direction. Want to appear with Christ in glory when He returns to set up His kingdom then accept Him as Lord. Declare the truth and live your life as a Christian. Don't conform and be buddies with this evil world.

When Christ appears we will be with Him in glory. Put to death you sins because wrath comes upon the sons of disobedience. Commit your life to Jesus and live in that new creation, redeemed and forgiven. Your eternal destiny is at hand and the consequence of rejecting Christ is too unbearable and it's an eternal judgement, not a gamble worth taking. Be strong in Christ by accepting Him as that final perfect sacrifice. Armor up daily by prayer, protect yourself against the devil looking to destroy you. Greater is He that is in you than he that is in the world. Stand therefore having courageously put on the breastplate of righteousness and act accordingly as you live within your new identity, Spirit filled cherished and forgiven, set apart as His family. Be bold for Christ. Intelligence is having a personal relationship with our Lord Jesus. Jesus was 100 percent God, the second person of the trinity. In Him was light. The world didn't comprehend Him. Jesus came to die and save those that were lost. His second coming, He will rule forever and ever.

"Not like a lamb, He'll rule like a Lion, change your ways or get kicked out of Zion." (Jeff Trigo, DC)

In His kingdom, all evil will be eliminated. With Him there will be no more death, no more sorrow or tears. One God, He became flesh. The Word became flesh and Jesus is the declaration of all that the Father is. Jesus is the full revelation of the Father. In Christ dwells the fullness of God. For your joy to be complete Jesus must remain in you and you must remain in Him. He gave Himself to sanctify us by His blood. The only authority that will rule forever in His glorious return is Christ. Spend time with Him in prayer and thank Him for salvation. Jesus our King, He is faithful and true, able to change people. Thank you Father God for Him, your Son.

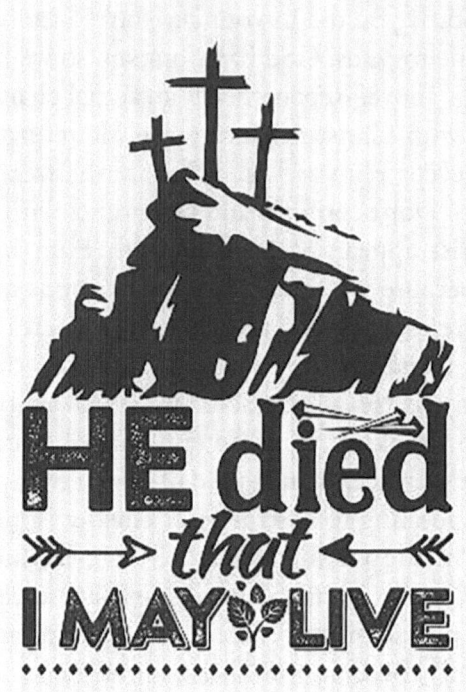

Jesus dwelt amongst us, put His eyes on the cross, died, and overcame sin. The power of Father God in Heaven raised His Son that third day. Your position in Christ is saved by faith receiving the gift of grace as God extends His mercy toward us which makes us a cherished member of His family, His Royal Priesthood. Sealed and indwelt with His Holy Spirit, our comforter and friend, whom will minister to you as which way you should go. This should secure you position in Him and solidify your mental health, we are already victorious in Him. The Cross did all that for you and me.

The faith which saves is not one single act done on a certain day: it is an act continued and persevered in throughout the life of a man. (Charles H. Spurgeon)

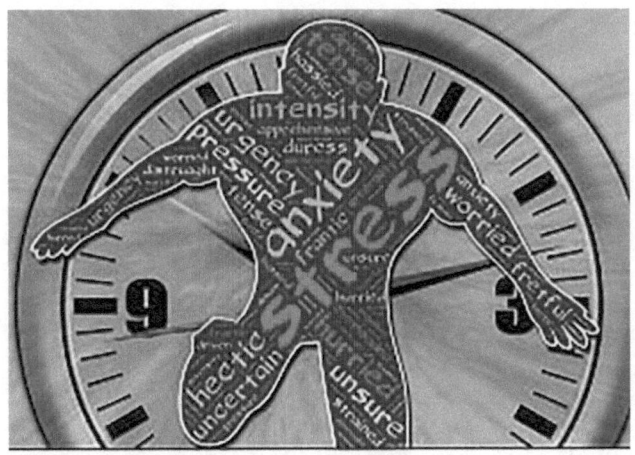

Worry: If we asked ourselves where is it that we waste time in our life, this topic of worry comes to mind, which by the way, only plagues Human beings. Take this good advice, its biblical, don't worry about the things you cannot change, and don't worry about the things you can change. If you can't change it then it's out of your control anyways, just pray about it and bring it to God; this allows Him to deal with it for you. If you can change the thing you are worried about, then do it and change. Worry causes stress and stress can kill. Stress makes you blood thicker and harder to pump while shortening your life. The more worry you give a topic or situation, the more it grows into that monster that controls you. Worrying is unnatural, unreasonable and shows zero faith. Besides does worry change the situation? No. It just messes up today doing nothing for the future. God feeds the birds of the air and they don't worry. We are in His family, created in His own image therefore how much more should we trust a loving God and worry less. Pray more, praise more and serve more and watch the worries of this world fade away. Stay on purpose with your goals and remember to follow through, that defines the super-successful, awesome follow through skills.

**"Whoever confesses that Jesus is the Son of God,
God abides in him, and he in God." 1 John 4:15 NKJV**

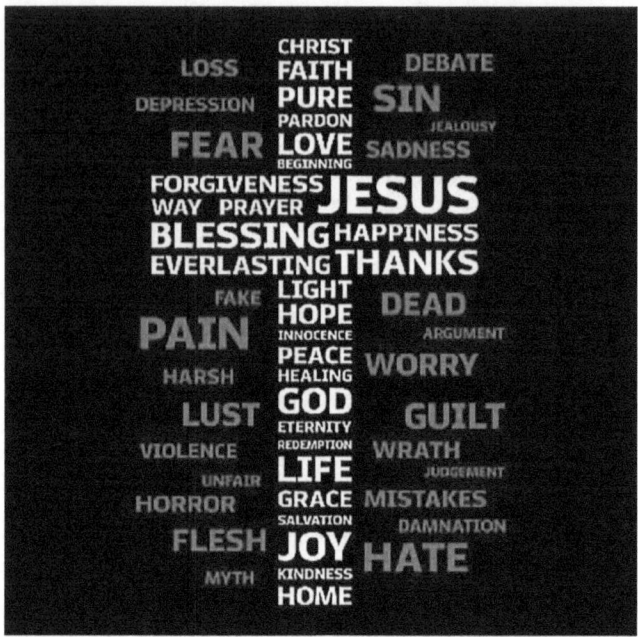

Self-Image: You can remember this one truth, that we are a forgiven people in Christ therefore learn to forgive others by also extending them that same grace. Learn to forgive yourself so you can start feeling victorious. We have an eternal passport to Heaven; therefore don't accept the enemy's bombs on your self-esteem. Sometimes I am my own worst critic, ease up and live in grace. Stop the self-ridicule, let go of regret, sorrow, anguish, pride and other joy robbing lies as you keep casting grief upon self. Live in faith, redeemed and forgiven. To the proud give them the law, to broken you give them grace. Fall in love with your core beliefs and let them be reflective of who you represent. We serve a mighty and loving creator, who desires to have a personal relationship with us. A Christian is a lifelong work as a sinner who through the refining process becomes a better representative of Him that is in us, toward being more usable for His purposes and His kingdom expansion.

**"Do not be wise in your own eyes; Fear the LORD
and depart from evil." (Proverbs 3:7)**

Are you being accused of being a Christian: If so, good, for out of the mouth come the desires of the heart therefore think before you speak and serve a bigger purpose than self! Always remember that your words can build up or tear people down. We are bombarded with negative thoughts and influencers all around us everywhere we go. Rise above and keep your eyes, heart and mind on heavenly thoughts considering eternity in ever decision you choose. Love more, compliment people more, help others, forgive often, let others know how much you value their friendship and keep your eyes on Jesus. By doing so, you will love the person you see in the mirrors reflection as the Holy Spirt takes up residence in your life feeling safe and comfortable and at home in your heart. You are an overcomer and a champion in Him, so enjoy your every breath and moment; in the end, rejoice, heaven awaits you, child of God.

Why I am here: We were all created to have a personal relationship with our Abba Father God in Heaven. Sin came into the world and separated us from a Holy God. The redeemer came to save that which was lost. This better covenant that He would send Himself as that final sacrifice, our kinsman redeemer, the chief cornerstone that was rejected, was Jesus Christ Messiah. Sin also created free will. By this freewill, we have the option to choose to worship by faith the one true living God, or make a fatal error and ignore the love story of redemption, thus be held accountable for your sins and face judgment day. I don't want to be judged, do you? I sure hope not, I would much rather be forgiven by grace receiving mercy because of faith in the finished works of Jesus on that cross. Invite the Holy Spirit into your life today. Pray to God the Father and ask Him to forgive a life filled with sin. Accept that Jesus brings you back from the lost and welcomes you into Gods family, forgiven by the blood, sealed with the Holy Spirit, God in you, an outreach of His Holy temple, a blessed and forgiven saved people. This breeds mental health and stability for eternal life, Amen.

Jesus said, "And you shall love the LORD your God with all your heart, with all your soul, with all your

mind, and with all your strength, this is the first commandment. And the second, like it, is this: You shall love thy neighbor as yourself.' There is no other commandment greater than these." (Mark 12:30–31)

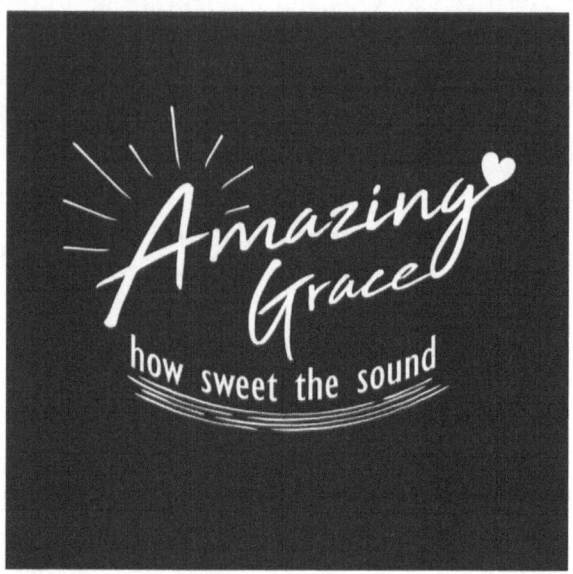

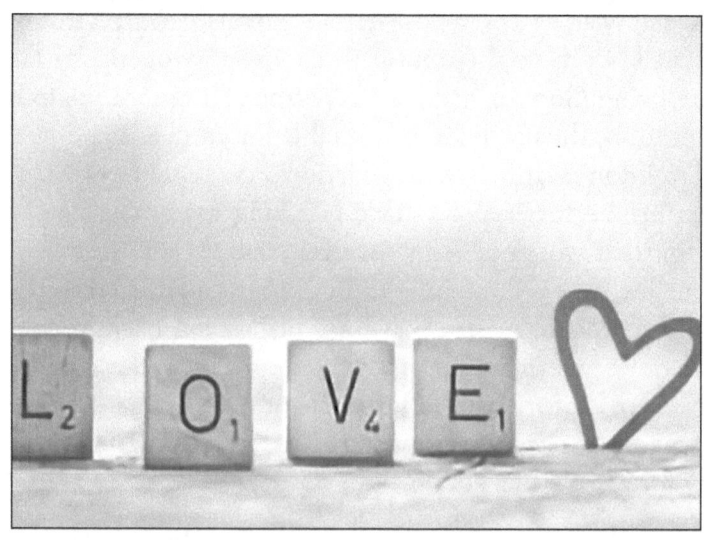

CHAPTER 11

Athletic Edge

When I was in Chiropractic College 1996-1999 we had a guest speaker come to our campus. I don't remember his name, however he was the chiropractor for the New York Giants professional NFL team. The story I was about to hear was a jaw dropper. Keep in mind I was a greenhorn and freshman in chiropractic school. Today, however 25 years later, when I reflect back it makes so much more sense. Players were getting adjusted in the locker room and getting over their ailment or injury fast. These athletes would be excited to get back on the practice field and when their physical therapist and other health care practitioners saw them walking by their station and on their way out to the field they would comment "it's time for your therapy session" and a common response amongst these NFL players was, "I already saw the chiropractor and I feel great, I'm heading out to the practice field" refusing other procedures. This made the other trainers feel insecure and that their job positions may be threatened therefore they had the chiropractor fired. Fired because his treatment was too successful? Wow.

"Fall in love with taking care of your body, mind and spirit, but don't forget the spine!" (Jeff Trigo, DC)

Today 32 NFL teams use doctors of chiropractic; I see tents that the players will go into after a hard impact or collision, hidden from the public eye, where a chiropractor adjusts the spine and/or limbs immediately thus limiting the effects of inflammation and reducing recovery time. Mostly all professional sports team employ a chiropractor on staff and those that don't should because their athletes may suffer career ending injuries that could have become asymptomatic if chiropractic was applied. Most surgeries will sideline the athlete for months, adjustments get you back in the game. You see, not only can athletes benefit from chiropractic care, we can all benefit. The adjustment will help the injury and/or prevent injury because a well-adjusted spine can take a better impact versus a locked and crooked spine. The adjustment improves recovery time from injuries, while improving the athlete's range of motion and strength. Chiropractic adjustments will create faster reaction times, improved circulation as well as general overall health while optimizing athletic performance.

Athletes that Utilize Chiropractic: Aaron Rodgers (his dad Ed Rodgers, DC, is a chiropractor), Arnold Schwarzenegger, Barry Bonds, Brett Hull, Charles Barkley, Dan O'Brian, Dan Marino, Derrick Rose, Don Sutton, Emmit Smith, Evander Holyfield, Fred Funk, Gerald Wilkins, Jack Dempsy, Jerry Rice, Joe Montana, John Smolz, John Stockton, Jonny Damon, Lance Armstrong, Mark McGwire, Maurice Jones Drew, Michael Jordan, Muhammad Ali, Rick Fox, Robert Parrish, Ronda Rousey, Scottie Pippin, Terrell Owens, Tiger Woods, Tom Brady, Venus Williams, Wade Boggs, Warren Moon, Wayne Gretzsky...

> **"As long as I see the Chiropractor, I feel like
> I'm one step ahead of the game."
> (Tom Brady, New England Patriots)**

I apologize for the great athletes that did not make my list, there are too many to name here. I just want the masses to see a very small percentage of the great athletes that utilize the great chiropractic healing powers. I wish I had the ability and time to name all the great stars in the entertainment industry, as well as professional teams whom employ chiropractic healers to tend to their precious assets, maybe we can start hearing them thank us on stage when they score or receive awards. After all, we chiropractors work hard behind the scenes to keep them returning to field or movie set for your TV/motion picture/slam dunking viewing pleasure.

"I definitely try to get on a basis where I use chiropractic at least twice a week. I would say definitely that is helps me to perform at a higher level." (Emmit Smith, Dallas Cowboys)

As athletes train daily, increased stress is put upon the spine therefore causing elevation in forces that can knock the spine out of its normal position. This regular strenuous exercise that creates subluxation causes unimaginable torture to the athlete thus even possibly ending the career too soon. Chiropractic care is a game changer to the athlete. Because of this noninvasive natural healing method, they can continue in the athletic arena without having to live with pain or get addicted to opioids. After all drugs are not good for your body and popping pills ignore the cause while creating harmful side effects that may hinder the athlete's peak performance. A numerous amount of injuries respond to spinal corrective care and a well-adjusted spine is stronger and more capable to withstand injuries upon impact. I have adjusted thousands of athletes and witnessed incredible healings.

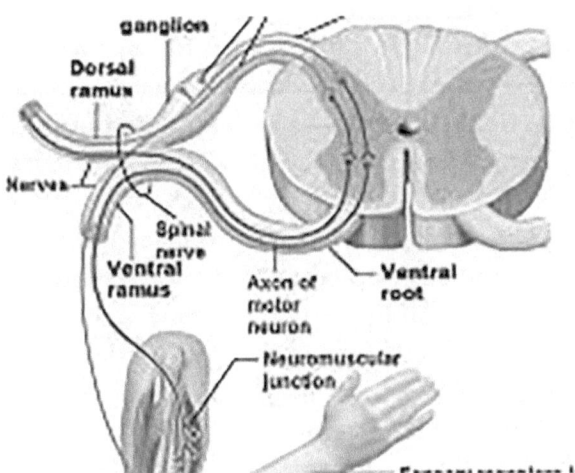

Muscles are 100 percent controlled by nerves: When a pinched nerve is present, the muscle that gets its innervation (nerve supply) is compromised and its ability to contract is lowered. This results in weakness, tightness, spasm, twitching loss of normal range of motion, etc. Postural distortions can also compromise the muscle tension with that being considered it is not the massage that's needed but the removal of the pinched nerve caused by subluxation and the biomechanical improprieties corrected. Sometimes a massage may make the bone more adjustable, but please don't lose site of the cause. Literally hundreds and maybe even thousands of patients have come in for shoulder issues. Many have visited after MRI studies were performed which suggested possible rotator cuff tears as diagnosis. Others after a series of cortisone shots, and some even presented post-surgical. One thing in common was that they all had a missed diagnosis of C5-6 subluxation. No one is looking to the spine for the cause of the ailment. The elephant is in the room and being ignored. In fact many different doctors point to different areas on the MRI as the cause of shoulder injury, not even able to agree on the actual pain site that is causing the symptom. Most of them are told it's a tear, or a cortisone shortage in the body. Stop the madness and get adjusted as a first line of defense not a last. We must have proper joint motion and nerve supply to be able to thrive. Only the well-seasoned doctor of chiropractic has mastered the ART of VSC correction.

> **"I didn't know how much I could improve until
> I started seeing a chiropractor. Since I've been in
> chiropractic, I've improved by leaps and bounds both
> mentally and physically." (Michael Jordan)**

I have a very strong male surfer athlete, Jerry age fifty, who couldn't even do one push-up because of a weak shoulder. Five visits later he is back to his full upper body routine, pain free and strong. He is back in the water surfing again where he feels most comfortable. Athletes benefit from chiropractic care because the results are fast and pinpoint the location of the problem. Training can be resumed without any long periods of down time and this can give the athlete the competitive edge they need over the competition that is not getting adjusted and trying to recover from injuries without chiropractic care. Low back pain is what ends most careers for the athlete and chiropractic care is 100 percent the treatment of choice for this. Remember the adjustment it's not a slamming movement or a twisting movement, but an adjustment to move the backward displaced vertebra forward and off the nerve. It's always safe, gentle and accurate, isolating one specific locked or fixated segment of the spine.

"I've been going to the chiropractor for as long as I can remember, it's as important to my training as practicing my swing." (Tiger Woods)

Concussion: Impact to the head or a violently shaken spine is the primary cause of this head trauma. Brain swelling may or may not be present, however the usual symptoms are headache or brain fog, difficulty with concentration, possible unconsciousness. Memory may be compromised, other symptoms include nausea, vomiting, fatigue, vertigo, confusion, sluggish response times and speech difficulties. Rest is a very important immediate helpful antidote, however if these concussion sufferers don't get their brain stem region adjusted, that is not good! Misalignment to the upper cervical spinal region, as explained in detail in chapter 5, causes brain stem compression on the spinal cord and make any other future impact more and more serious. If you have experienced a head impact of any kind at all in your lifetime, then go see a chiropractor ASAP. The preferred X-ray needed to evaluate this misalignment is called a A-P open mouth Nasium view with a 5 degree cephalad (up wards) tube tilt. A qualified professional, a.k.a. the chiropractor, could then analyze the occiput, C1 and C2 positioning and then take his/her highly skilled hands to make the necessary corrective adjustments. These adjustments will fine-tune and realign the spine back into its proper position so innate wisdom can function most optimally again. Love the hands of a gentle healer with the gentle corrective touches, a.k.a. adjustments, removing nerve interference and restoring function. Expect miracles because each day is a new day for healing and it's never too late to start chiropractic. Maximize your wellness with the health compound effect by starting care as early as possible, the younger you start the better the results. All subluxations will cause the spine to rot away, it just take about 2 decades. Please don't let this happen to you or someone you love, chiropractic awareness is of paramount importance.

"As a professional athlete, I am highly competitive-only accept the best. When it comes to healthcare, chiropractic is an essential service. It keep my on-field performance at its highest level and contributes to the success of the entire team." (Reggie Bush)

With concussion care, make sure you are icing the neck region and stay hydrated, drinking plenty of water, fish oils, creatine, and rest during the recovery period. Use turmeric in the diet more, fresh pineapples and other natural anti-inflammatories. Slowly ease back into your exercise program with post-concussion care. Remember the all-important adjustment and rest period. Anti-oxidants help aid and support all of the brain functions and restore the elastin stretch components of blood vessels, so always take them regularly for maximum benefits. Hyperbaric oxygen chambers will aid in recovery time and provide that little edge on your way back into the "big game"!

"I did a lot of things to stay in the game, but regular visits to my chiropractor was among the most important." (Jerry Rice)

"The job of the chiropractors is to restore balance, symmetry and function. This will maximize innate wisdom to flow effortlessly." (Jeff Trigo, D.C.)

"When stress and conflicts arise, losing your cool is not an option!

Trials should make you better not bitter. Faith leads
to obedience which sparks action and strength
with Devine guidance". Jeff Trigo, D.C.

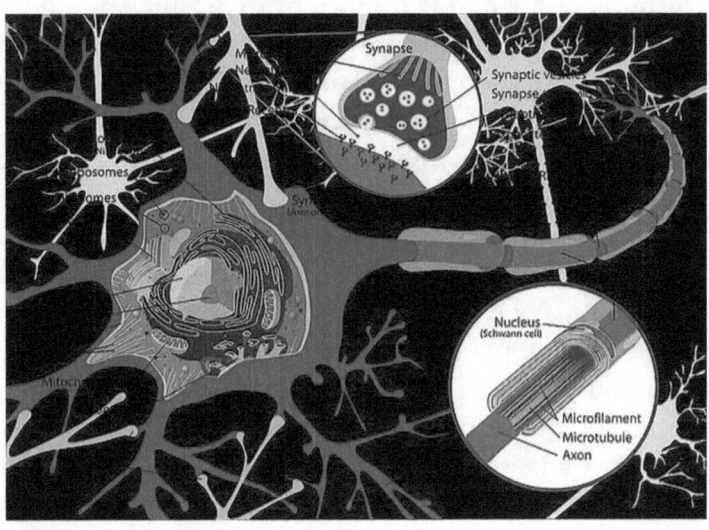

Fact Check: If a muscle is completely dependent on proper function of the nervous system and athletes depend on their well-conditioned bodies to perform and react at levels well above the average human beings capability, then pinched nerves caused by subluxation will limit athletes from reaching their maximum potentials; It makes sense to seek spinal realignment adjustments to correct subluxations that all spines inherently get during this journey called life. Life, full of physical forces like bending, twisting, stooping, slouching, falling, poor posture, slips and falls. Add athletic insults: collisions, tackles, repetitive injuries, twisting, swinging, wrestling, pulling, pushing, lifting, landing, flipping, hitting, slamming, crushing, kicking, etc. Also add in a mix of chemical and emotional forces; we all get subluxations, it's inevitable. The competitive edge in an athlete is so important, and so is winning! Subluxation will rob you or the athlete of physical power and hit you right between the eyes while affecting your mental power as pain pours into an unstable foundation, linked to a kink of a nerve, limiting greatness. Feeling busted, get adjusted. Don't pout, your spine is out. You bend them we mend them. Truth.

"Performing at my best is important to me and should be to everyone. I am blessed that my dad is a chiropractor. Getting adjusted regularly-along with practicing other good health habits that my mom helped me to establish—are all part of my goal to win in life and on the field." (Aaron Rodgers)

Regular Adjustments: As an athlete, every second counts. Having that athletic edge means the difference between first place and seventh. Nutrition may be the fuel to the body, which is so important, but without nerve supply you are dead in the water. It should now be clear and logical that chiropractic is not opinion, but fact. When properly applied expect injuries to recover, pain to dissapear, numbness to regain sensation and the reversal of arthritis as motion is restored. Healing takes time and prevention is key. Regular visits will prevent the need for prolonged healing times necessary in cases with chronic neglect. Don't forget, a strong and well-adjusted spine increases the load in which it can withstand in regards to impacts and forces.

The toned muscular system aids in reducing the frequency of subluxation while aiding in support and strengh of spinal integrity. A force of impact on the adjusted spine is easy to absorb via its natural free flowing spinal curves hence preventing injury. The adjusted athlete will recover faster and will absolutely experience a diminished injury time while maximizing a long successful career.

"Dedication sees dreams come true." (Kobe Bryant)

The only concern of the athletes should be to focus on winning. That athletic edge becomes compounded when we see an incorporation of a wellness lifestyle into their daily and weekly habits. Nutrition, exercise, practice of their craft and proper preparation become the building blocks towards greatness, however one must include spinal health in order to gain a long career and aquire that edge needed to become a champion!

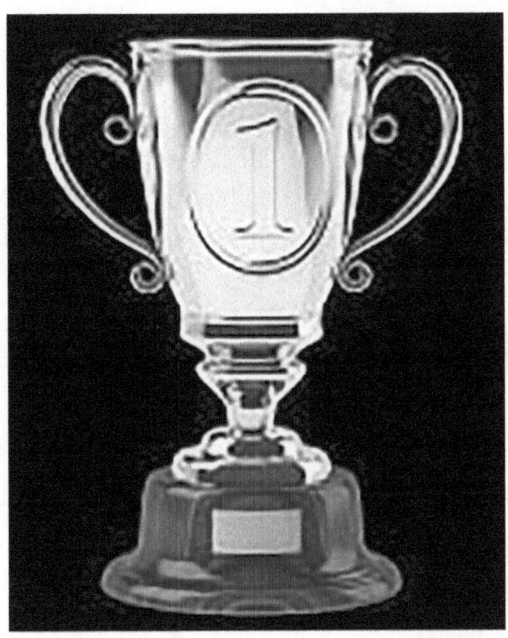

Without chiropractic care: The athlete like all vertebrates, will experience the subluxation effects. The pressure on the nerve will show up as some sort of symptom ache or pain. The joint starts to dry up within 2 weeks, but continued movement by the athlete is actually causing a dry disc to start to rip, tear and rupture. Disabling conditions are lurking and ready to show its ugly self as disease or disability and symptoms suddenly start to appear. Muscles start to guard and ache while weakness begins to appear. Reaction time and strength are reduced. Athlete starts missing games, due to subluxation being masked as some type of condition misdiagnosed as tendonitis, bursitis, or other aches and syndromes. Real cause undetected and misdiagnosed. Posture distortions worsen and clamped nerves shut off function in organs, tissues, cells, glands, muscles, and areas of the skin. Symptoms get chased as cause is ignored. Endless therapies procedures and pills are dispersed upon the person with subluxation as causation remains intact. Expensive tests are all negative as they are not looking to the spine for the cause and prevention of disease as quoted by Hippocrates. Money is spent treating symptoms that are all being caused by a spine with VSC, and the athlete continues to get all sorts of treatment but is not offered or given a corrective adjustment. The team starts to lose because of your absence, they draft for another player and you're cut from the team, losing your ability to make a living and pay the bills. All because you ignored spinal maintenance and have never embraced the fact that all spines get subluxations. Don't live in "Subluxation Denial", every spine matters. Gravity will subluxate your spine so get it aligned!

"The moment you give up, is the moment
you let someone else win."
Kobe Bryant

This book will change anyones possible dis/eased future into a wellness journey. Prolong your abilty to compete and stay in the game. It's my hope that all woud not be fearful but educated in the importance of spinal tune ups, a.k.a. adjustments, to correct vertebral subluxation complex, and start winning again. Adjustments save lives, save careers, save finances, and save marriages.

Hyperbaric Oxygen Therapy: Today's athletes have so many different tools available to help them obtain and maintain the competitive edge. In today's insurance industry many conditions have been accepted by that will now authorize payment for services in a hyperbaric chamber. The 60 to 90 minutes that will be spent in the very open highly compressed oxygen chamber will benefit your health in so many different ways. The oxygen saturation while under a pressurized environment aids in the formation of new blood vessels thus increasing blood delivery to areas that were subjected to inflammation, trauma and/or poor wound healing. Concussion patients that get adjusted and undergo hyperbaric O2 therapy have amazing short recovery times as they get over their brain fog quicker and this recovery can be observed in their athletic performance. Any person with a brain injury, poor wound healing, carbon monoxide and cyanide poisoning, diabetic patients with gangrene, bacterial infections, can all benefit with hyperbaric oxygen therapy. This will reduce dependency on pain killers, stimulates osteoblast and osteoclast (bone and cartilage forming cells) can also benefit from this treatment. Hyperbaric treatment has also shown improved brain activity in post stroke, alzheimer's and dementia patients. Benefits also included the treatment of diabetic ulcers, improvement of hearing loss, anemias, provides an environment in which cancer can't thrive, aids in fungal and bone infections, helps in the recovery of radiotherapy, aids in the acceptance of skin grafts, treats liver injury and heart disease. Reduces cancer and tumor growth and aids in treating seizure disorders. Helps scuba divers to recover from the bends. This therapy shows to mobilize stem cells for tissue regeneration, while reducing the risk for amputation and resolving diabetic ulcers.

More and more benefits are being released to the public as studies continue showing that natural treatment methods like this one that can only help you with no risk of harm in anyway. I am a fan of natural healing methods, not harmful shady practices that have poor results and life ending side effects.

The well-tuned athletes need to use all they can to fine-tune their divinely created bodies to maximize performance while obtaining and maintaining that competitive edge.

"If you don't believe in yourself, no one will do it for you." (Kobe Bryant)

CHAPTER 12

Children Are People Too

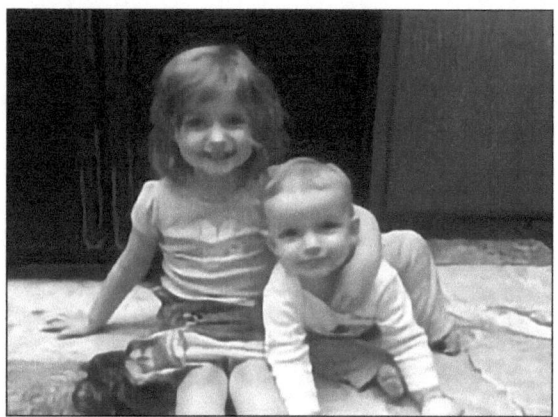

Gianna and Dante, adjusted since birth.

But Jesus called them to Him and said, "Let the little children come to Me, and do not forbid them; for of such is the kingdom of God." (Luke 18:16)

A child is such an innocent pure little soul that's full of life. Wonderfully made and designed to last 120 years but yet totally dependent on others upon arrival. Where is the parent manual to teach the proper raising of a child? To ensure the child is raised with love, good character, integrity, forgiveness, mental strength, hope, courage, faith and so forth. Teach them how to problem solve, and to communicate in a loving tone. At the earliest age possible get their spine checked, teach them about real food and hard exercise. Finally to graduate them into adulthood, a rite of passage they deserve. A child must be given the chance to be as healthy as they can possibly be and not altered via outside-in medieval medical intervention like injectable toxins and pills that are forced upon them at earth's arrival. These toxins have shady and awful side effects that cause a change in their wellness destiny thus slamming them toward dis/ease, autism and autoimmune disorders! Let them have a chance at life as created and wonderfully formed in the womb. Stop the test tube, and laboratory scams that changes the child's wellness into a life altering, dis/eased and symptom filled future via M.D. interventions. What happen to that voice, a voice with freedom of choice that demands the release of these harmful ingredients contained thereof for scientific due diligence so that each ingredient contained within may be looked up and with informed choice can a parent then consent or decline said blood chemical Russian roulette cocktail. Anyone can have a child, this section of the book is to shed some light on good parenting skills which I believe should be incorporated into the expectant parent's procedure, a mandatory class on parenting. This chapter is not a class but it is full of gems and wisdom which should help to contribute to many healthier and happier well adapted thriving children worldwide.

> **"Whoever causes one of these little ones who believe in Me to sin, it would be better for him if a millstone were hung around his neck, and he were drowned in the depth of the sea." (Matthew 18:6)**

Play Time: Kids need at least 1 hour per day of daily physical activity. I suggest 2-3 hours for better physical fitness levels. This includes good old fashion outdoor fun like running, climbing, swinging, monkey bars, chasing, biking, swimming, etc. The physical fitness aspect of life (see chapter 8) with kids is paramount as they go to school, interact with their peers while gaining confidence in their own abilities. Physical activity will not only keep the weight down but also enhance their mental capabilities. Light contact sports should be encouraged when they start showing an interest, and eye hand coordination skills developed by playing games of catch and throw will help them with many other life endeavors as they embark upon the athletic realm. Green zone, is considered time outdoor with nature like hikes, exploration, camping, etc. This is also needed on a regular basis.

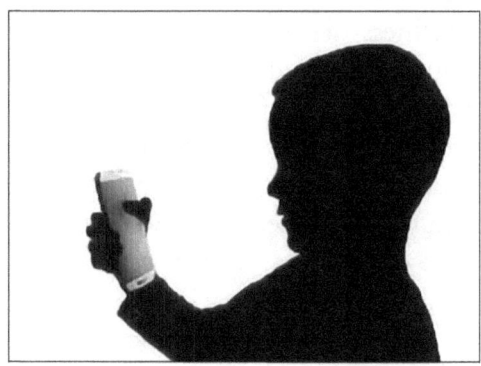

Screen Time: The TV or video game is not your babysitter. Kids are spending too much time in front of the TV nowadays. The average kid spends close to 7 hours a day in front of the screen. It's no wonder that there is an epidemic of child obesity in America today. Kids older than 6 including their parents should have a maximum screen time of 2 hours a day. Spend the rest of the time in books, arts and crafts, board games, sports, puzzles, learning an instrument, etc. As the physical fitness and playfulness time increases in the child's schedule, you will notice more of a welcomed desire for the child to want to go outside and play with their friends.

"If you can't feed a hundred people then feed just one." (Mother Theresa)

Communication: I love getting down on one knee and looking eye to eye into the eyes of my children. I'm not towering over them and forcing them to look up, but at eye level for some great eye to eye interaction; feels much safer to the child. Another parenting skill I like to incorporate is for a minute instead of in a minute. Dad will you come over here and help me with this? Or, dad can you play with me? I like to say, if I'm super busy, for a minute instead of in a minute. Then go, connect, have fun and enjoy them while they're young, they grow up fast. A communication skill set of being a good listener and not their problem solver takes time and practice to master. Encourage their feelings and reinstate the obvious when they march in very frustrated at a certain incidence: "wow Johnny, you seem very frustrated with your sister right now" Jane can you see how frustrated your brother Johnny is?

How can we create a win-win scenario that satisfies both of you? Allow the children to problem solve and figure out who goes first and for how long and who goes second for possibly longer as a benefit for waiting. Set clear understandable limits. "I have to set a limit and not allow you to hit your sister, this is over stepping the boundary of keeping a safe space between the two of you." If you yell at your kids, your kids will also yell at others. Tone is everything! Even the best advice will get ignored if the tone is uncomfortable to the ears. Want to be heard, keep the message and the tone in alignment with your heart and the message will not fall upon deaf ears. This takes practice and you will only get better at it.

> **"A man's wealth is not measured by monetary figures, but by the number of his kids, children are the crown of His glory, on loan to us from above, God loves them more than we ever could." (Jeff Trigo DC)**

Unique: A child's personality and their love will shine forth, and as a parent we need to learn how to observe and absorb the unique personality that this little soul possesses. Watching children play and allowing them to decide what they want to do, explore or play with, creates wonderful bonding moments and opportunities for the continued positive growth of the parent child relationship. If their blocks are stacked up crooked and is bound to tumble over, let it. Saying you need to do it like this, will not teach them anything. They need hands on learning; the hand-eye coordination and problem solving skills are hard at work here.

This child also needs to feel important and special. Remind them often of that, they will appreciate it and it further instills thrust for you within them. When your child speaks to you, listen to the conversation, don't just rush them off because your agenda is too filled with tasks that are of less importance, your child is more important. Get animated, get on that knee, be interested, and interact. I also like to let them be involved in the decision making process. Give them acceptable options regarding restaurants, movies, parks, activities etc., and be ok with their choices. This will make them feel powerful and important to you. Let them know what an awesome valuable family member they are thus creating that sense of belonging. Hold their wants and desires in your mind and keep them engaged in a two-way communication highway that is safe and without judgment. Explain the consequences of their bad choices or behavior and allow them to make informed choices thereafter.

Most importantly, always smile at them, be gentle, hug often, create bonding moments daily and love them unconditionally.

"If you then, being evil, know how to give good gifts to your children, how much more will your Father who is in heaven give good things to those who ask Him!" (Matthew7:11)

Divorce: God hates divorce. With that said, regardless of the drama that ended the marriage, shield you children from the drama as much as possible. A child should never have to hear one parent complaining about the other parent. They are innocent bystanders that are getting hurt and experiencing stress in this divorce also. Failed marriage is more common now versus in the last 20 years, a prophetic end time's prediction. A successful marriage takes 2 imperfect sinners to possess great levels of forgiveness and love. It must be Christ centered, and you put the need of the other over the need of self. It's biblical.

"Nevertheless let each one of you in particular so love his own wife as himself, and let the wife see that see respects her husband." (Ephesians 5:33)

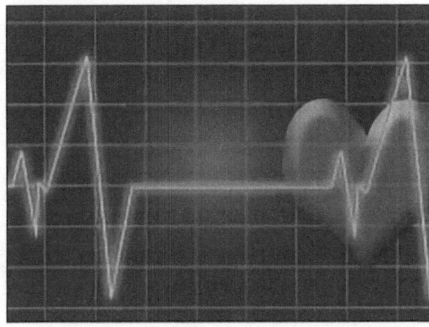

A successful union consists of a 3 stranded rope: Jesus, husband, wife. Couples that pray and read the Bible together, stay together. Any breakdown it that three-way relationship often brings divorce and a divided home as their kid's parents part ways. Chalk up another victory for Satan who loves to attack the marriage as this leads to a child's innocent heart to become broken. Fight to save your marriage. Remember what it was in the beginning that created the union in the first place. The grass across the street is full of weeds, you just can't see it from your own home. Love one another and compliment often. Celebrate all of your important milestones. Never stop dating your spouse. Give at least 2 daily compliments to your husband/or wife telling them what you appreciate about them. Communicate-communicate-communicate! Forgive often and love without holding back. Unfortunately people will continue to get divorced, it's big business in America, and the lawyers are the only ones who really benefit! With that said here are some simple rules to help the children in this horrible process and new dynamic that was suddenly heaped upon those letter shoulders.

Rules to follow in broken homes:
Children that have been subjected to divorce have certain rights that must be followed. We owe it to them.

- To be treated as important human beings, with ideas, desires feelings and an important team player. Having a sense of belonging.

- The child's right to a continued relationship with both parents, if a safe, loving and secure environment is being offered at both locations. The kids need to feel safe expressing love towards both parents.
- The divorce is not their fault, make sure they know this and you can never tell them that you love them too much.
- A child's voice is always welcomed and heard with love, withholding of judgement, while plenty of guidance from both parents is encouraged.
- A child can freely express love and what they appreciate about the other parent without being silenced, judged, manipulated or reprimanded.
- A child has the right to equal access to both parents on a regular basis (50:50) if both locations offer a loving, safe, healthy environment.
- The children should always have a relaxed feeling while in the comfort of their home that we are providing for them.
- A child should never hear a parent badgering, ridiculing, complaining, or talking bad about another parent.

"Husbands, love your wives, just as Christ also loved the church and gave Himself for her..." (Ephesians 5:25)

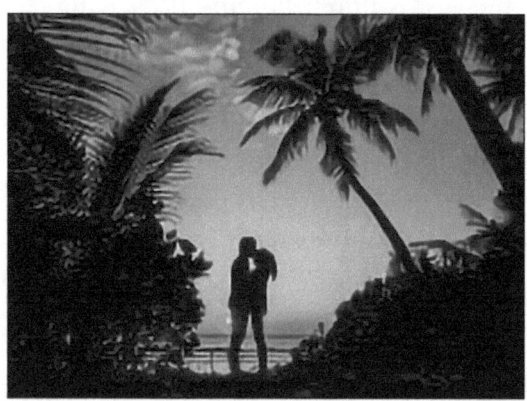

**"Wives, submit to your own husbands, as
to the Lord." (Ephesians 5:22)**

Chiropractic for Children: The birthing process is hard enough for the mother and the child, which will absolutely produce subluxation on both spines involved, but then we get to add another statistic: kids fall on average 1500 times by the time they reach their second birthday. Kids need gentle accurate spinal tune ups also. Many health problems that can be witnessed through infancy, toddler stages, even adolescence and adulthood, can be traced back to tiny structural changes in the spinal positioning caused during the birthing process and manifesting itself as symptoms showing up at any time and even up to a decade later. Chiropractic adjustments have helped infants suffering from colic, digestive problems, ear infections, vomiting, tonsillitis, and many others symptoms. Children that get sick often or have asthma like symptoms, achy joints, neck tilts, shorter or longer limbs, popping sounds in their spine, fatigue, falling a lot, growth pain, or other health concerns must first have their spine checked by a chiropractor before trying a cocktail of harmful medication that treat the symptom while ignoring the cause, pinched nerve via subluxation. As children embark upon their physical education time, sports, etc., the need for chiropractic care increases while also providing an increase in coordination and peak performance. While chiropractic care is vital for the whole family, the regular check-ups can prevent minor injuries from becoming major ones. No matter what your child's age is, chiropractic tune-ups will make a huge difference in their wellbeing. It is so important to check that their natural healing capacity is functioning at optimal levels to ensure they obtain the maximum physical ability that they are capable of achieving.

**"You have brains in your head you have feet in your shoes you
can steer yourself in any direction you choose." (Dr. Seuss)**

Please steer your family in the direction of a healthy proven success and wellness option by choosing chiropractic as a first line of defense and prevention and not as a last resort after the regimen of pill popping, surgery and other invasive procedures. Babies, get adjusted, children get adjusted, I take care of 90 plus year olds and they not only see improvements in their everyday activities, they return again and again for the soft gentle healing touch that awaits them at my office, you can too.

"Don't delay, get adjusted today." (Jeff Trigo, DC)

"Don't let anyone tell you that you are not perfect and try to add a toxic pill for completion, you were made in Gods image, therefore let your sparkle shine." (Jeff Trigo, DC)
"Have we traded mumps and measles for cancer and leukemia?" (Robert Mendelsohn, MD)

Injectable Substances: We must ask ourselves why, we as a nation of people, continue to believe a lie thus, continued allowance of a toxic mixture of Frankenstein's potion of the season; something to inject into our bloodstream, bypassing all our normal portals of entry (nose, mouth, lungs, etc.) and have direct interaction with our organs, glands, cells, etc., without any real solid evidence that doing so will do more good than harm! Then have the money to bribe whoever they need to make it pass as law to really boost profits while igniting sickness sales at your local pharmacies. Where is full disclosure of ingredients with proven results of health benefit absent any harmful "side effects" or DNA damaging results? The public has the right to review the laboratory cocktail ingredients and make an informed, educated decision on whether or not they want it injected into their precious child's perfect bloodstream. No such ingredient label exists my friends, it's all a corrupt way to start the sickness downward spiral that brings in big profits with big sales, as the sickness business executives cash in on your illness.

"Chiropractors detect and correct the cause of nerve compression and interference, allowing your body to self-regulate, adapt and heal. Get your whole family checked for VSC ASAP." (Jeff Trigo, D.C.)

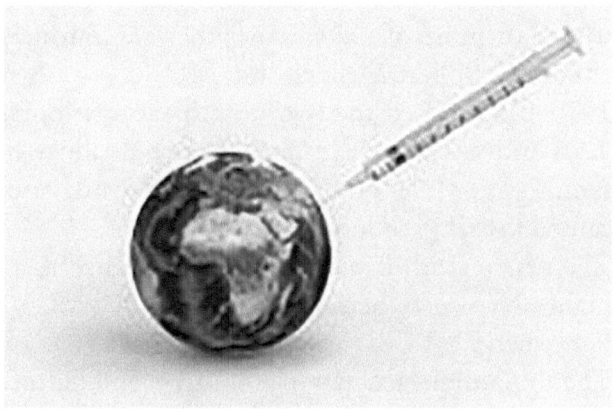

**"Do nothing from selfishness or empty conceit, but
with humility of mind let each of you regard one
another as more important than himself; do not merely
look out for your own personal interest, but also
for the interest of others." (Philippians 2:3–4)**

Did you know that in many studies written by various doctors of
all degrees and areas of health and science professionals (MDs, DCs,
PhDs, institutions, US government, collegiate studies, and others),
have collaborative studies that all confirm the following results when
vaccinations are giving to the child:

- Research shows that non-vaccinated children are healthier
  than vaccinated children.
- It has shown to be a very rare occurrence for non-vaccinated children to get all the problems we see in vaccinated
  children like: Autism, auto immune disorders, ADD,
  learning disability, dyslexia, immune system compromise,
  behavioral disorders, mental compromises, neurological
  disorders, etc.
- "My suspicion, which is shared by others in my profession,
  is that nearly ten thousand SIDs (sudden infant death syndrome) that occur in the United States each year are related

to one or more of the vaccines that are routinely given to children." Robert Mendelsohn, MD.

- 1975 Japan raised the two-month vaccination age to two years and saw a drop in incidence of all above mentioned symptoms while going from seventeenth most deaths caused by SIDS to lowest in the world.
- The person with five consecutive flu shots has a ten times higher chance at getting Alzheimer's according to Hugh Fudenberg, MD.
- The unnatural vaccination is invasive and harmful to your baby while breast milk boosts immunity and resistance to pathogens, etc.
- Outbreaks have occurred in population controlled environments I where 100 percent of the people got vaccination yet many still get sick anyways.
- Vaccinations in childhood have been linked to cancers according to Robert Mendelsohn, MD.
- Vaccinations have been linked to damaging the participant's DNA which opens Pandora's box for a whole realm of sickness and disease
- Immunizations against common childhood disease have caused us to trade measles and mumps to leukemia, cancer, autoimmune disorders, Asperger's disease, Gullain-Barr syndrome, eczemas, encephalitis, meningitis, seizures, deafness, and many other diseases that also include problems with normal digestion, eye, ear function, comprehension, and more.
- Polio was on the decline (95% eradicated) when the vaccine was introduced to the public. This was due to the implication of sewage systems and hand washing practices; there is no proof that substantiates otherwise.

What Is In A Flu Shot? If we are truly free in America then how is it that political bureaucrats can pass a law allowing all children in the public system to have mandatory poisons injected into their blood stream prior to enrollment? It's not working and doesn't protect our kids from anything! In fact it bombards our children with toxins overloading their poor systems causing them more harm than ever. However if you are a pharmaceutical company or peddle drugs in the sickness arena, then it makes sense to bribe lawmakers into making this unscientific scam, thus making it law. Did you know that the number one cause of measles is the vaccination which spreads the disease? Let's go ahead and examine what is really in a flu shot:

- Mercury, a neuro-toxin. In 1999 the government asked to remove this chemical but still it persist in many flu shots today. Mercury has a great attraction for brain tissue, liver cells, bone marrow, digestive track and kidneys. Symptoms of mercury injected via flu shots are 100 percent linked to Autism.
- Formaldehyde, another poison, except this one has been linked to causing cancer, a.k.a. carcinogenetic properties. Also linked to leukemia, reproductive harm, respiratory complications, and other immune compromises.
- Sodium deoxycholate, allows for tumors to grow and breaks down the integrity of DNA.
- MSG. a neurotoxin that also causes birth defects and reproductive harm.
- Gelatin, associated with allergic reactions.
- Sodium Phosphate, causes lifelessness, GI compromises and is a neurotoxin.
- Polysorbate 80, has been shown to cause cancer in animals.
- Neomycin Sulfate, inhibits the uptake of B6 therefore allowing for mental retardation, and epilepsy, allergic reactions and other life-threatening conditions.
- Chicken embryos have exposed allergic people to chicken or eggs causing them to become seriously ill.
- Beta propiolactone, known to cause harm to organs in multiple places.
- The preservative Thimerosal contains mercury, linked to causing autism.
- Sorbitol, linked to GI disorders.

- Octoxynol and its derivatives, is a spermicide, causes toxic reactions anywhere in the body and should never be considered as an injectable.

ADHD: Effects 2.5 million children in our schools today. Exercise, sugar elimination and chiropractic have shown to be effective in the increase of math and reading scores in children with ADHD. Exercise is a safe alternative to harmful drugs and more cost effective. We preach keeping the schools a drug free zone yet will give our children a weakened form of horse tranquilizers? Educate, don't medicate! Limit their screen time and have them do plenty of physical exercise. They are perfect in design and don't need outside in (drugs/injectable etc.) influence. Let's take a look at some triggers to avoid and some helpful natural remedies to aid the precious children that suffer from ADHD. Remember that this book is all about the non-invasive drug free approach to healing and when it comes to your children, they are worth the effort.

> **"Parents are the ultimate role models for children. Every word, movement and action has an effect. No other person or outside force has a greater influence on a child than the parent." (Bob Keeshan)**

For children with ADHD: Here are 16 helpful tools for you to implement:

1. Avoid preservatives and food coloring—they trigger symptoms.
2. Keep your child away from potential allergens.
3. A diet rich in B vitamins, zinc, L-carnitine, and minerals like magnesium, calcium, etc.
4. Plenty of exercise and outside time in the green zone.
5. Get plenty of fish oils in the diet, avocados and other essential omega 3-9's. The child can eat wild caught salmon for this, tuna, sardines, etc.

6. Ensure proper gut health via probiotics.
7. Natural raw foods are high in nutrients and are needed in proper development.
8. GABA is a calming amino acid and can help sooth your child.
9. Turkey has tryptophan in it and helps regulate production of serotonin for proper sleeping cycles.
10. Keep them drug free, please.
11. The single most important thing you can do is to avoid sugar.
12. Regulate proper sleeping habits and make sure your child is not sleep deprived.
13. Develop great communication skills so that the children will feel safe to communicate what's causing them to become frustrated, angry, etc. A useful tool in small family groups is to pass a "who's turn to speak" toy or object that is soft and fluffy. Tone is everything! Use lots of I statements.
14. Take a step back before an attack. In other words retreat and think about what needs to be the loving tone and message before you react.
15. Allow fidgeting, it's a good steady release of energy. It can be made less with physical activity, stress balls, fidget spinners, rolling of 2 marbles in one's hand/or coins, etc. If you kid fidgets relax, its soothing and will not hinder any learning according to available research on the web today.
16. Teach your child to make a list of 20 things to do and 3 things to be. This will help them to stay focused, enhancing memory and help them in the areas they need improvement.

"Train up a child in the way he should go, And when he is old he will not depart from it." (Proverbs 22:6)

CHAPTER 13

"Big Pharma"

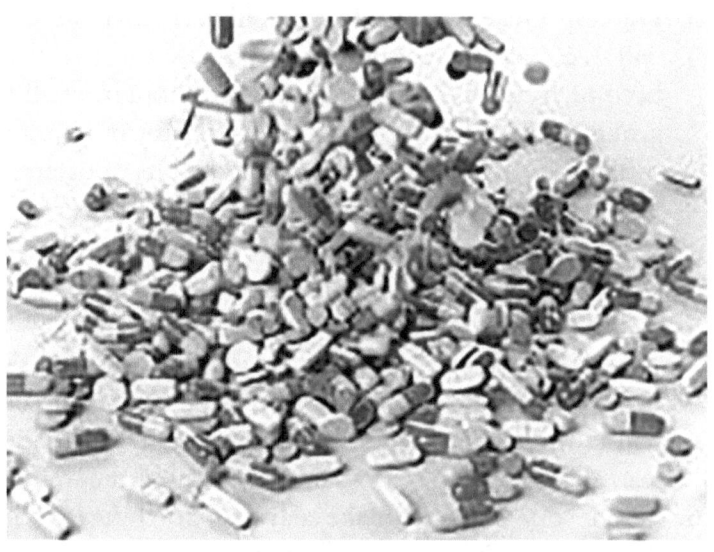

There is a sickness story told by millions with its many variants, tweaks and twists. It's very common in my country, and is reaching pandemic proportions. John Doe has been suffering from headaches so he picks up some aspirin at the drugstore, he is hopeful in seeking relief. He has noticed a decrease in headache intensity but is curious about what to do with these new ulcers burning stomach pains showing up. To the store he goes looking for ulcer relief meds. John Doe has received some heartburn relief but notices if he doesn't take the medication then symptoms return so he continues and as a few months pass, he has noticed some bouts with unexplainable diarrhea, dizziness and respiratory infections, body aches, cough and/or chronic fatigue. Confused about what to do next, he gets told by the doctors that an antiviral flu/colds medication should be taking. Upon taken this new medication which now includes NSAID's, he feels like fainting, worsen dizziness, low sperm count, tinnitus, lower sex drive, and diarrhea with continued chronic tiredness. Occasional nose bleeds are now happening after one month's passing and some real concerns are now apparent as John Doe steps on the scale and sees double digit weight gains from chronic pain and lack of gym involvement. His mental status is now in a state of depression and despair. He now was asked to pick up an anti-anxiety anti-depression medication to cope with this new life changing mental state he suffers daily with. Guess what, John Doe is now losing his sex drive, and has broken out in rashes. His heart has arrhythmias (irregular heartbeats), pink eye has shown up and has been diagnosed with a new thyroid condition and has been suggested to start taking thyroid medication ASAP.

I can continue adding to John's downward spiral story but I would really rather not. This is a vicious cycle that is immensely terrifying while being great business for sickness care and good profit for drug companies while having nothing to do with wellness care. This is just another gross mismanagement of the patient's health while ignoring the atlas, C1 subluxation, as headache causation in the first place. Americans are in pain and they are spending over $3.2 billion every year on over-the-counter drugs alone, not counting those available by prescription. 18 billion was just for pain relief. The opioid epidemic has cost Americans more than $500 billion since 2001, and is expected to cost us another $500 billion over the next 3 years. According to http://cdc.gov/drugoverdose/epidemic 91 people die every day due to overdose of prescription painkillers.

Chiropractic adjustments, healthful eating and going to the gym are a much better choice. Stop playing Russian roulette with your health. Each pill has a handful of side effects that continue to show up needing the next outside in (pill) lie to swallow. Remember health is an inside job. Reset that circuit breaker first and watch the intensity of neuro-electrical impulses from the brain to the tissue cell return to normal levels reversing dis/ease while restoring joint motion and lubrication by this safe inside out approach, ADIO, via chiropractic adjustments.

> **"Any man can make mistakes, but only an idiot persist in his error."**
> **Marcus Tullius Cicero**

Health doesn't come in a bottle or a syringe, and the person on the most medications is not the healthiest. The opposite is quite true. We are an accumulation of our daily actions and habits we developed over a long period of time. By the time they reach 60 in America, 20 percent of the public is taking at least 5 different medications; 9 percent were taking more than 10 medications. Not me, not my kids, not in my house! In fact if you don't take any medication at all then you are now amongst the rare minority. I am happy to say that I belong to this group (living in the med-free zone) and I didn't even fill the prescription to get pain meds for oral and hand surgery, or pain meds for a broken rib I suffered in 2012, didn't need it. They only fog your brain's clarity while creating constipation (loss of peristalsis) and slowing down your body's metabolism thus healing takes longer. Besides do these pills know to go to your right distal second phalangeal area on you hand? No. Better off with ice.

Your pharmacist, or local drug dealer—all a matter of your perspective, may not catch dangerous drug interactions that happen when drug combining starts. It's not only the side effects of drugs you have to be concerned with, but when drug combing starts, you have to worry about the side of the side of the side effects? In the USA 2,000,000 adverse drug reactions (ADR's) occur every year in which 100,000 people die. This is now in the top 5 most common ways to die in America! This has to STOP. No thanks, I won't be in that statistic of people who died from sickness care.

"Did you know that side effect is a made up term? In Science, we have cause and effect, not side effect." (Jeff Trigo, D.C.)

Studies conducted by the Institute for Healthcare Informatics now called Quintiles IMS, revealed that $200 billion a year, or 8 percent of the US health care spending, is spent on medical care resulting from improper or unnecessary use of prescription drugs. From 1997–2016 the amount of prescriptions filled in the US rose by 85 percent despite the population only growing by 21 percent. The FDA calls ADR's "a significant public health problem that is, for the most part, preventable, noting that cost associated with the care needed for ADR's is $136 billion dollars a year. You also have a 1 in 5 chance of being injured or killed if you are in a hospital due to ADR's. America change the way you think about sickness care now, and start focusing on wellness. B.J Palmer would say, "change your thots." You are intelligently designed, lacking nothing. Get adjusted and turn the power on! That pill needs to be a last resort, not chiropractic. Change your perception; embrace the wellness concepts taught in this book, and visualize that life you want, not only symptom-free but a life full of vigor and spunk. MD Tool Kit: 75 percent of all doctor visits end up with the physician giving the patient a drug prescription. I find that to be malpractice. Do no harm. If a patient can get better with a gentle corrective adjustment instead, exercise or proper diet changes then why would they want to put a patient on an endless drug dispensing regimen? Most drugs they are dispensing are being pushed on them from local sales pharmaceutical representatives that really have not had long term exposure and adequate testing for ADR's. According to the FDA, a drug will be released to the masses only after 1500 patient exposures, which may not be enough to detect serious risk to the patient. They also wrote, "Some drugs cause serious ADR's at very low frequencies and would require many more exposures to detect the reaction." Wow, I hope this has got you thinking! There has to be a shift in the way we view our human design. You have options to choose, consider these 2 choices:

Popular Choice: Flawed and imperfect; are you sick? Add drugs and procedures please. This is the "out-side-in" theory, AKA "germ theory." Example you come in contact with something outside of your body. This germ or virus gets inside of you and you become sick. Therefore you need to take this outside pill and put it inside your body to get healthy. Horrible results causing millions of deaths. This choice leads to big profits from sickness care and harmful shady results that often make you worse.

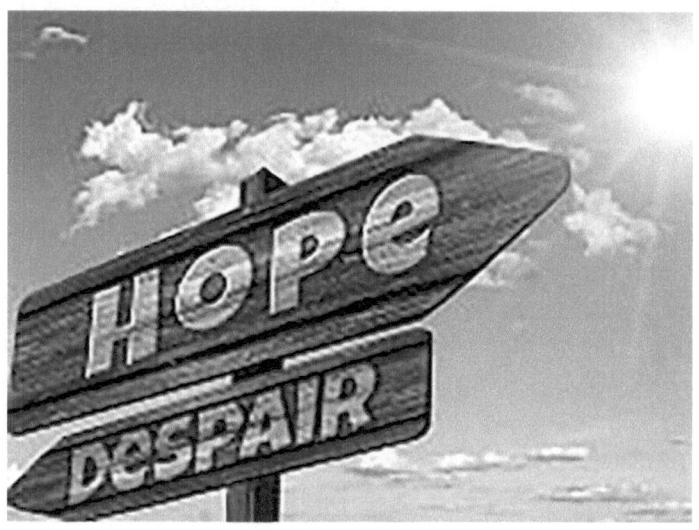

The Minority Choice: "Inside out" theory. Humans, a perfect design, created in His own image. The nervous system, travels from the brain above, down the inside of the spine and out to all organs, tissues, glands, muscles and cells of the whole body. Life flows no other way. A well-adjusted and subluxation-free person will still get that germ or virus exposure but the immune system is optimized thus killing it fast. For example, a sinus working with 100% nerve supply doesn't sinusitis. What a profound concept! Have an overload of a food poison, or digested a toxin, the body will rid itself of it, detoxify it, digest it, kill it with a fever if necessary, remove it by throwing up, etc. It can pick and choose whichever function and method it needs to deal with this health invader as it deems necessary. After all, the immune system is also controlled by nerves. You see a well-adjusted spine will allow its nervous system to do anything it needs to as long as there is 100 percent innate wisdom operating at 100 percent of the time. Lifestyles can include healthy eating habits and exercise as a mandatory conjunct. But this type of lifestyle is where you will find the happiest healthiest people in the communities. They don't get sick as decades pass. They are not carted off to the ER for a sudden clogged artery. This is due to healthy preventive eating choices compounded over time. You won't find them in a drug prescription line. They are the active thriving healthy minority that chooses to have no nerve interference and are living in the drug free zone, perfect in design, absent toxicities and deficiencies. Remember, even conjoined twins who share the same bloodstream get sick separately, it's not germs, otherwise they that share the same blood would get sick at the same time! Different levels of VSC exist on them thus causing a loss of function at the involved level of the spine. We can observe above-down-inside-out working at optimal levels in the adjusted patient. Feel free to look up the Russian girls Masha and Dasha for yourself, they shared the same bloodstream but yet expressed different symptoms of dis/ease. God doesn't make junk and we are not weak. The fact is we don't need all of these laboratory chemicals that create more harm than good. It's not science!

"Then God said, "Let Us make man in Our image, according to Our likeness; let them have dominion over the fish of the sea over the birds of the air, and over the cattle, over all the earth and over every creeping thing that creeps on the earth." (Genesis 1:26)

Most medications dispensed are from multiple MDs and these drug pushers do not always consider what medications you may have already been prescribed thus really increasing your risk for ADR's considerably. In a Chicago investigation of 255 US Pharmacies, it turned out that dangerous drug companies are putting millions of American lives at risk representing an "industry failure." 52 percent of the pharmacies investigated handed out drug combinations that could result in stroke, kidney failure, oxygen deprivation, unintended pregnancy, birth defects and other dangerous health risks.

The actual warning about dangerous ADR's were not being given and voiced to the public. Pharmacists were not notifying the patient's doctors about adverse reactions that patients were receiving after being prescribed these dangerous drug combinations, and simply stamping a sheet of paper to the bag was not acceptable because most people just throw that paper away. Software designed to flag potential interactions doesn't exist and after seeing so many of these red flags pharmacists were glazed over and immune to these warning signs thus failing to inform the patient. Talk about a flawed and broken system in which people are the Guinea pigs.

More Drugs Taken, Less Life Expectancy: The average life expectancy continues to fall in America with the latest results that were obtained in 2015 putting the US average life range at 78.8 years. Much lower than Europe and Asia countries which range from eighty to eighty-four years. Even Cuba had an average life span of 80 years. The reason for this lower age upon death should be obvious by now. But to put it bluntly, the opioid epidemic, chronic mismanaging of disease and dysfunction, obesity, and unhealthy life style choices, over medicating doctor practices, exploratory surgeries and failure to offer healthy alternatives are the primary reason. Despite that fact that health care costs in America exceed 3 trillion dollars, we are one of the sickest nations ranked "worst performing system" by multiple aspects of care. Wellness is not an option with these pharmacists, and the doctors who are dispensing these drugs are not offering natural healthy remedies as options for the public which has, to a fault, put way too much trust in these shady practices. Big changes are needed and I need your help to make this book go viral.

If you would, please take a picture of this book and post it on your social media sites; you can tag me, and I will also share it. Join my Facebook group: To Heal A Nation. Please share that also. Together we can make a difference! Dear Father God in Heaven, thank You for Your divine design in creating us, Your people. Thank You for Jesus, His holy sacrifice; and by faith in Him, we welcome Your gift of the Holy Spirit to indwell us, guide and protect us while teaching us all of Your Holy ways. You are a God of abundant love, hope, mercy, and grace. We are lucky that You, our Father, desires to have a relationship with us! We as a nation lift up the wellness concepts taught in this book and ask You to allow wonderful healing throughout our great land. We are thankful for all You are doing in our lives, and we look forward to the positive changes we will soon see in a wellness community. In Jesus's cherished name we pray, amen.

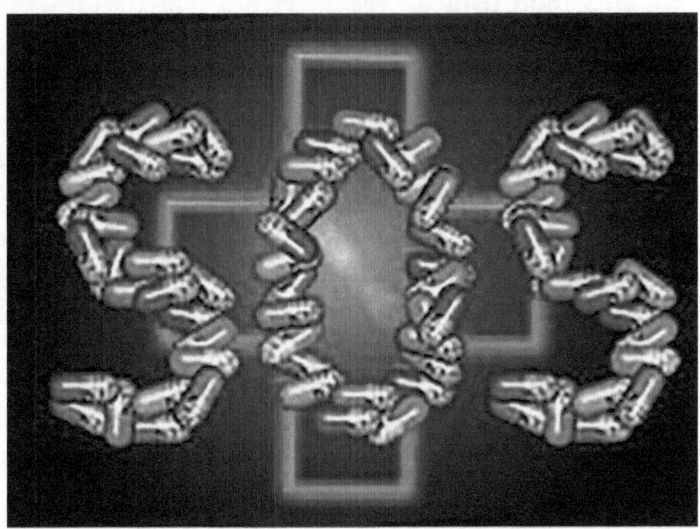

Opioids: I want to start this chapter off with a moment of pause-reflection of all the lives lost to this deadly drug.—Say a prayer for our Great Nation right now and ask that we create a change in the way we take care of our lives and how we manage pain. Wellness must be taught. That's the only way to change the path we are on.

We must apply the concepts taught in this book first before pain drugs. Please pray for our great nation and the people thereof now. In Jesus's name we pray to our Father God in heaven, amen.

Oxycodone is one of the culprits, but Fentanyl is the opioid that is the most common in drug overdoses. It's a synthetic opioid and is responsible for an increase in deaths annually between the years of 2013-2016. In that same period this pain killer is responsible for 63,632 overdose deaths. Including my brother Peter. As a comparative example, a jumbo jet plane holds approximately 550 passengers. 63,632 ÷ 550 = 115.69 plane crashes in 36 months killing 63,632 people, that like 3.21 jumbo jets falling out of the sky monthly, would you fly? I wouldn't. In 2012–2015, heroin killed fewer people at 15,961.

In 2017 the over prescribed opioids have been in the news and making headlines. Not for any good reasons but because of the 70,000 people that died, more than any year on record. This dropped the average lifespan of Americans to an all-time low of 78.6 years. This problem is apparently unique to America only. The USA accounts for only 5 percent of the world's population yet it consumes 80 percent of all the opioids. Why are Americans in so much pain? The medical mind set likes to dispense drug to the residents of America versus finding and fixing the cause. The elephant is in the room, stop ignoring it. It's called subluxation, as a result, this crushed nerve, which is very painful, is one of the main culprits of the pain syndromes we are plagued with. Go get adjusted and remove the most common source of pain and dis/ease which is VSC. Cost of an adjustment on average is only $50.00 bucks.

To make matters worse: "Big Pharma" spent billions on marketing physicians to promote opioid sales, including offering physician's perks like vacations, dinners, cash incentives, etc. In areas where opioids were marketed we see a higher death rate versus the areas that were not targeted. JAMA observed this link between physician-forced marketing and increase in opioid-related deaths and 400,000 different marketing payments for doing so! Criminal actions indeed, don't you agree? We have MDs acting like drug dealers, we should prosecute accordingly.

America needs to stop spending 3 trillion dollars a year on these shady practices. Rich pharmaceutical companies getting fat off of the countries' demise is unacceptable, we the people of the United States of America must demand a change. Most medications are a result of bad and unhealthy lifestyle choices which could have been avoidable in the first place. Be an example, put down the soda can, put on your gym clothes, get that body moving and sweat a bit and most importantly, go make an appointment with the chiropractor to have your spine evaluated for VSC masking as some other dysfunction or health riddle. Imagine what Americans could do with an extra 3 trillion dollars, while being the healthiest place to live and setting an example to the world. No longer being led like sheep, but with a change of "Thot" on how we approach wellness care, we as a nation can heal by the billions. Move well, eat well, think well and live well.

Drugs are never the answer and medications don't make you well, they are drugs. Wake up citizens of earth, where's your fight? Take back your health and demand wellness care not sickness care. There is no quick fix or magic pill folks! Take accountability and change your activities of daily living. Remove all toxic eating and toxic behaviors while addressing all necessary deficiencies that may be present like lack of chiropractic, nutrition, physical exercise, JOY, prayer, contentment, etc. Stay in the present, let go of the past, focus on what you have to do today to be the healthiest version of yourself, and never take your eyes off your goals. Jesus wants you to be healthy and succeed, give Him the glory by praising and worshiping Him.

Pharmacy: There are 2 different methods in which drugs will hit the market and become available for the public consumption:

1. Corporate venture capitalist—These tycoons investors buy old drugs and revamp them with a bunch of hype and market them as they launch forward seeking big profits without scientific backing—I'm not ok with this!.
2. Science base—Placebo controlled, double blind studies that are peer reviewed and scientific in their research—I'm ok with this in moderation, teach preventative lifestyles and apply all the tools and concepts that this book has to offer and eventually be living in the drug-free zone.

De-Prescribing and Detoxification Trend: Ask your doctor if the drugs you have been prescribed are actually healthy for you and curing you of original presenting symptom. The fact is that the drug is making you less healthy and not helping to cure anything. Be assertive and ask your doctor to show you how to get off the harmful medications you are on, how to detoxify your system and limit any harmful withdrawal symptoms that may be associated with discontinuing the swallowing of their pills and lies. Even the best medical schools are not preparing the doctor to heal patients adequately while finding the root cause of the problem. Instead there are trained to quickly prescribe medication, or do surgery and not to give the body a chance to heal naturally or offer safer alternatives like chiropractic, nutrition, exercise and other lifestyle changes. The whole sickness care system is rooted in maximizing their profits as opposed to helping people regain and maintain their health.

Reducing and eliminating these pills are your best protection from ADR's and often puts you in the fast lane back to wellness and health. Go natural and safe, change your lifestyles immediately and get on the wellness bandwagon. Live in the drug-free zone, often thriving in the green-zone while embracing the compound wellness effects.

"Chiropractors are obtaining results that I could have not obtained with medicine or surgery." (F. C. Rutherford, MD)

An ounce of prevention is worth a pound of cure. Stay regular with you spinal check-ups. Eat as healthfully as you can, stay active and exercise daily. Find a way to get off any prescription drugs, because there is always a safer more natural way to take back your health and live in a wellness drug-free zone that's subluxation free.

If you are willing to stay determined, work toward a detoxifying goal and keep getting back up after being knocked down, then you will be able to someday achieve all the health goals you want and create the life you have always dreamed about. God will finish the work He started in you, follow where He leads and leave the rest to Him. To obtain the success you seek lies in your ability to continually improve and fine tune your actions and activities of your daily living. Never give up and don't settle for mediocrity. Don't wait for a miracle, pursue your dreams 100 percent by doing your part to the best of your ability and capacity. Ask God to make up the difference. Take that leap of faith and God will act. Trust Him, trust prayer, trust the healing that begins when natural remedies are applied and if you lack any talent, then work twice as hard to make up the difference.

God heals yesterday and allows you to effectively live today. Let go of past regrets, and old unhealthful habits so that they don't hinder growth for the future. The blood of Christ forgives you therefore concentrate on building a new drug-free healthier and happier you.

"God gives each one of us the desire to soar. We are created in His image, which means we were not meant to creep. Fan into flame your highest ideals, your greatest God-given desires, and let them take wings. You were designed for the heights." (John C. Maxwell)

Finally, stop putting so much darn trust in laboratory produced chemicals, pills, potions, creams and chemical cocktail and shots that try to mask your symptoms while creating a whole new batch of unwanted new ones. Question everything and do more research if needed. Look up each prescribed medication for yourself and see if all those "side effects" are what you would desire for yourself. I assure you that this is not for you, and that there is a much better natural homeopathic way to obtain safer results. Seek natural remedies that have great outcomes and experience for yourself the quick natural return of wellness, absent of dis/ease and symptoms. It is my desire that those who read this book, take to heart all that is written within and apply its principles earnestly, without haste and live a thriving long life for it.

"Rescue me from my enemies, Lord; I run to you to hide me." (Psalms 143:9)

"Now to Him who is able to do immeasurably more than we ask or imagine, according to the power that is at work within us, to Him be glory in the church and in Jesus Christ throughout all generation, for ever and ever!" Amen. (Ephesians 3:20)

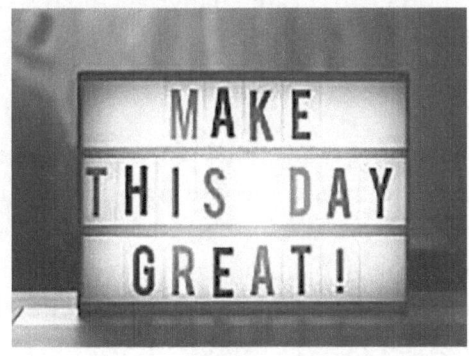

CHAPTER 14

Insurance Ideology

Insurance is big business in America today. Billions are spent on prevention of loss, and when it comes to health care, this number is absolutely astronomical! With that number in the hundreds of billions, why is this system flawed and broken? Why would insurance pay for sickness care and not preventative wellness care? Why would Workman's Compensation Insurance, a federally run program, operate at almost bankruptcy? Why is the great USA not so great at health and one of the unhealthiest countries to live in on earth? Our life expectance rate is lower than some third world countries! The Manga report, in chapter 7, sheds some light on the positive quick noninvasive results that were obtained when chiropractic care was implemented as a first choice "portal of entry" doctor in regards to the condition of lower back pain; the financial savings of the nation were in the billions. In order to create change in today's world, we must demand that insurances offer a different kind of coverage, wellness coverage. Teach wellness, breathe wellness and pay for wellness.

What is health: Absent of symptoms? No. Many people feel great and are symptom-free right up until they suffer a heart attack! The dictionary states: "freedom from disease" and in another translation, "the general condition of body or mind with the reference to soundness and vigor." I think we can improve on this definition, how about this one: The absolute 100 percent expression of Innate wisdom maintained by an individual who is absent of toxic chemicals and lacking zero deficiencies, while eating and training his mental, physical and emotional self toward an eternal perspective absent sabotaging lifestyles, decade after decade. That was fun. You get the big ideal by now hopefully. I've been hammering it home to you throughout the theme of this book. So, how can we improve the insurance industry, that gets rich off your premiums while paying for your sickness care and quick demise if you get too expensive to cover? Did you know that 80 percent of the bulk payments to doctors from insurance for your life long care is during the last stages of life?

**"Success is not a destination, it's a journey
and a process." (Jeff Trigo, DC)**

I mean really now, most doctors study disease therefore can never get the sick well, and it makes sense. You can't study the habits of the homeless to become wealthy and the same principle can be applied here, you can't study the sick to get them well. We must study wellness to get the sick healthy.

I believe that insurance should start paying for prevention, which is a much smaller fee, versus the huge fees for sickness care, invasive procedures and costly tests while ignoring the cause which is often pinched nerves, bad eating habits and sedentary lifestyles.

**"Chiropractic is health insurance. Premiums
small, Dividends LARGE! (B. J. Palmer)**

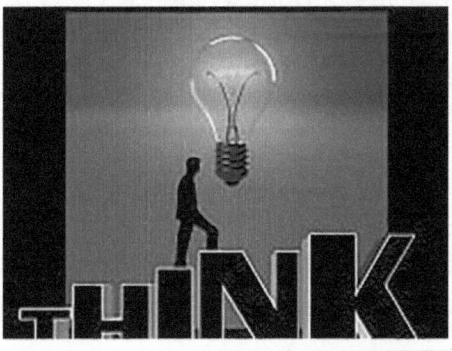

Gym Membership: How great would it be if your insurance paid for you gym membership and in order to keep it active, a minimum monthly attendance is required. Doctors could sign off on your out-door activities like the bike ride or jog you took, or that all day surf or ski adventure, etc. Maybe even document the exercise on a web site showing proof that you trained inside or outside the gym. The gym has an internet functions that logs your attendance and reports to the insurance company and the people who go most often get lower premiums. Yes it's a far-fetched ideal but we the people of the United States must start to unite for a greater and healthier America. This will also prove you to live better and longer because those who visit the gym with regularity seem healthier and more agile than those who do not.

"Treatment without prevention is simply unsustainable." (Bill Gates)

Nutritionists: Another mandatory insurance requirement would be teaching people how to eat, and shop for healthy foods. Include cooking tips, portion size and so forth. This could eliminate diabetes, obesity, heart disease and more. Foods could be promoting life versus robbing you of it. Set up mandatory webinars that one must sign into and answer some easy Q and A's at the end. This will assure that the lifesaving educational information is doing what it's supposed to do, reach the masses, increase their wellness IQ while lowering the cost of sickness care as a result of eliminating decades of junk food consumption and their poisons, clogging artery effects, dyes and pre-servatives and their contribution to a shorter life.

Poor eating habits can cause plaque to build up in the vertebral arteries, Chiropractors know how to test for this and know how to safely deliver a lifesaving low force cervical adjustment to remove your suffering. Don't be fooled by a pill pusher who states "don't get adjusted" they are clueless to our methods! Chiros know when to adjust and when not to.

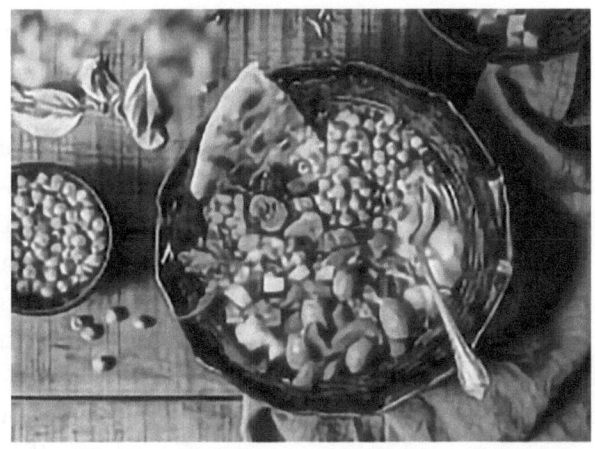

"Healing is an inside job." (B. J. Palmer, DC)

Dentist: Another important part of health care that is generally under paid for by insurance companies is dental care. It is no great secret that we need to take care of our teeth, tongue and gums. Unhealthy gums can spill bacteria into the blood stream and their favorite spot to find a home happens to be on the heart valves. Not ok, get yourself a water pic and add that to your brushing and flossing regimen that includes brushing twice a day and include your tongue. New products available include a non-rinse bone forming toothpaste. This will reduce the amount of damage caused by bacteria eating away the enamel. Remember to floss and rinse often. Increase in insurance coverage for dental care will create healthier, happier smiles across America.

"Research found that people with gum disease are almost twice as likely to suffer from coronary heart disease."
(American Academy of Periodontology)

Problem Solving: One could ask now, how can insurance cover more of the wellness cost while costing us less out of pocket money and not go broke in the meantime? We must look at the bigger picture here, people no longer have diabetes, no longer have back and neck surgeries, asthma, IBS, vertigo, high blood pressure, etc. They implemented the tools of wellness and millions of surgeries like carpal tunnel, shoulder cuff scams, sinus jobs, spinal fusions, etc., are all disappearing. Billions of dollars are no longer being spent on pharmaceuticals, opioids, procedures and death. There is so much money left over now because America is getting healthy and wealthy, sick days are a thing of the past, work productivity is up, students are learning better and we are living in a healthier nation now. It happens day after day, spine after spine, bite after bite, jog after jog and town to town, that's how we do it. B. J. Palmer, DC, talked about this with his "big ideal." We stand united, one wellness voice! Now there is a plethora of money left in the insurance companies' bank accounts to be able to afford to cover a small monthly gym membership fee, seasonal dental visits, weekly chiropractic adjustments, nutrition and cooking online classes, etc. Put wellness care before disease care! Prevention before symptoms!

Chiropractor: God Bless Rosa Parks and her movement to the front of the bus. I've stated it many times that chiropractic is the "Rosa Parks" of the health care industry, however it's also the best hidden secret to obtaining fast healthy results to free you of your symptoms. After chiropractic was slammed by the AMA (chapter 7), for one hundred years; it's no wonder there is a stigma hangover in the air. I even have to ask my patients to bring the insurance checks in to me because sometimes the checks get mailed directly to the patient and not the chiropractic doctor, what a shame that is! Do you think that insurance companies are doing that to their local MD drug dealers? Also Medicare patients will get coverage for their care only if the chiropractor is a provider and their secondary coverage is denied. Medicare is not accepted? That's discrimination folks! Only the Chiropractor has to fight for his worth and the adjustment is the most important healing entity that turns the body's natural healing powers back to the on position for normal neurological function while simultaneously restoring motion in the joint which as you now know is vital for the nutrients ability to flow in and out of those areas promoting life and longevity for the spine. Insurance must pay for chiropractic, this is paramount, and not 6, 12 or 24 visits! It should be on an as needed basis with a minimum of 1/week, 52 visits a year! There would be plenty of wellness money available to afford this preventative health-care service. Wellness is on the rise and sickness has reached its demise.

Subluxation Denial: Well it is about time we clear the air folks. We all get subluxations whether you believe it or not! You have learned about our vital nerve energy that gets switched off with that silent killer called subluxation. 100 percent of the time it will lower innate wisdom by diminishing proper nerve flow. You understand the importance of regular joint motion and the arthritic conditions that follow all locked joints. 100 percent of the time a normal spinal segment will rot away within 2 decades maximum if VSC remains present. With that new found knowledge, will you demand better chiropractic coverage for every member of the family? 52 visits a year! We are talking about small gentle accurate adjustments that fine tune innate wisdom and flip the power back on; 365.25 days a year living with 100 percent nerve supply and joint motion. What will you do with no more sickness stories; tell health and wellness stories while living in abundance and excellence?

You found the cure to health and it doesn't come in a bottle, it's our daily choices that we are making and they can really add up over a lifetime. Move well, think well, and eat well, because you only have one human life to live, therefore make wise choices that are in alignment with your goals and desires.

> **"If I'd known that I was going to live this long I'd have better taken care of myself." (Eubie Blake)**

Trauma Coverage: It makes a lot of sense to have insurance plans that can cover traumatic events because accidents do happen like: car collisions because too many people need to look at their phones instead of the road, don't drive intextacated or intoxicated! Falling out of a tree and breaking a limb, sports accidents, slip and falls, etc. This type of coverage is accessible when applicable toward the insured individual. After the initial fire department response, time to call the carpenter to fine tune your body. Remember that the fire department and hospital is for the traumas but not for general wellness with their drug addiction tactics. The carpenter, a.k.a. chiropractor can now reposition that bent frame of yours and assure proper nerve and joint function and get you back to preinjury status. Failure to visit the chiropractor may result in lifelong symptoms that get worse and worse while robbing you of your life and wellness. Then you get prescribed more and more lies that chase symptoms all over the body and surgeons suggest more and more cuts and procedures, especially if insurance will pay for it, no more please! Stop this flawed way of thinking and embrace change. Seek out that which is good and will do you no harm, safe and natural, with proven wellness results.

"As the hammer looks for something to strike, so the scalpel seeks something to cut." (Jeff Trigo, DC)

Health Crisis Coverage: Unexpected cancer, brain or bone tumor, stroke, etc., that is what this insurance coverage is for; however, please keep in mind that the principals in this book when applied, are very preventative for many of these conditions and when implemented at the earliest age possible, we should see a tremendous drop in the number of these cases therefore saving millions of dollars for the insurance companies while improving the health of the nations! Prevention is much more effective and affordable while being in the best interest of the patient.

Uninformed Public: Because of the lack of great chiropractic insurance coverage in the market today, thousands of people want to go to a doctor that is covered by their insurance. They miss a healing opportunity and settle for some lesser treatment thus ignoring causation, subluxation, toxicities, and sedentary lifestyles. Why would the public let their insurance company dictate who they get to see for care? Often there is a young employee say age 22-25 on the telephone line dictating who and when you get to see a doctor and the public is ok with that? Just because insurance may pay for that shot, potion, lotion, pill, bolt or screw, ice pack, electrode, therapy session, blue goo etc., that doesn't mean that is what's best for you. Have you heard all options? Most chiropractors will accept a cash price that is similar to the copay of an out of network specialist as full price. We must demand better coverage and change the way we think. Chiropractic is more important than teeth brushing so no matter what is offered, take health matters into you own hands and control your own wellness destiny. Choose chiropractic, exercise, and nutrition always. Be informed, not a victim.

Privatize Insurance companies: Offer stock to shareholders that are the insured and are paid dividends for nonuse. Insurance companies will pay for the gym, chiropractor, nutritionists, and dentist while avoiding costly sickness care. The insured can qualify by taking a physical exam, fitness test, receive a clearance letter from the chiropractor, and pass the nutrition online quizzes, then you're insured. Quarterly or yearly dividends get paid back to shareholders, the insured people, as rewards for wellness and keeping costs down because they are healthy! Accidents happen, dental care, chiropractic care, gym fees, nutritional classes, etc. that is when insurance pays out. All treatments and the gradual recovery process are being done through noninvasive wellness procedures. This is wellness and prevention at its best. The type of care we can witness that will bring health to each home, town by town, county by county, state to state healing a nation. Pill popping has to stop if we are to become a great nation that has a healthy ranking. I don't know about you but I am sick and tired of being told that America is one of the sickest and unhealthiest places to live in the world. Change is possible and it starts with you.

"Dance with your fear until it turns into courage" (Chip Esajian)

www.chipesajian.com author of "The Victorious Mindset."

CHAPTER 15

Freedom of Choice

Choices exist all around us, should we go left or right, talk or listen, sit or go. Should I smoke or quit, act or wait, eat healthy and workout versus junk food and sedentary living like a couch potato glued in front of the TV or video games. Decisions can lead to many different paths, some towards health and success, while others toward disease and poverty. Endless surfing the internet and getting lost in all the content have caused people to lose their jobs or business due to lack of follow through skills. Others may have suffered potentially life changing consequences due to poor decisions. Sometimes the effects are seen immediately while others play out over time. That it is why we need to wake up praying and carefully consider every choice heaped upon us daily. All choices should have some common denominators when considering our options. Is this choice going to move me toward my goals or further away. Is the choice I am about to make in the nature of God, brings Christ the glory and is helpful and loving to others? Or is it self-serving, and always about self-centered motives. We can choose to live a life that keeps our thoughts as being heavenly minded (vertical relationship) or held captive and horizontal (earthly minded).

> **"If I take care of my character, my reputation will take care of itself."**
> **D.L. Moody**

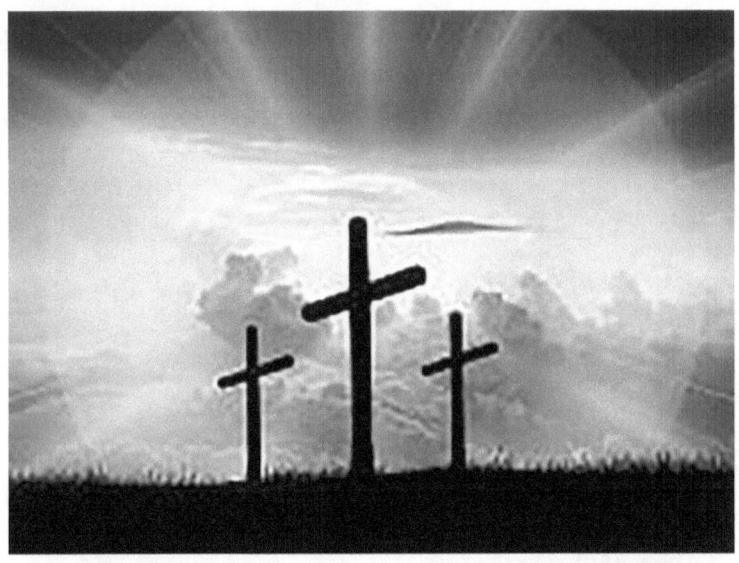

Church for God or Man: When choosing a church to attend many important factors exist but one stands out over them all, is Jesus the focus? Is this church a Bible teaching church or do they skip around endlessly with feel good messages? The best way to learn the Bible is page by page, book by book, and cover to cover. If your church is not a Bible teaching church then beware of wolves hidden in sheep's clothing. The message should be about the Gospel of grace and mercy as our Lord victoriously conquered death, a perfect and final sacrifice for the forgiveness of sin by the blood of our Savior, Jesus. If that is the kind of church you attend then the other factors to be considered: The children's ministry, missions available, community outreaches in place, areas in which you may serve and the body/congregation. If by the third time your attendance to church has not netted any friendships, research shows that people tend to move on to another church. So church goers, be friendly and say hi to strangers. A smile goes a long way, ask people their names, try to remember them and introduce them to others.

"Read your bible and pray, every single day." Jeff Trigo, D.C.

How much does our God love us? Wider than the universe, higher than hope, and deeper than death! (Pastor Bert Almazan) A very profound statement! www.CalvaryBeachside.com

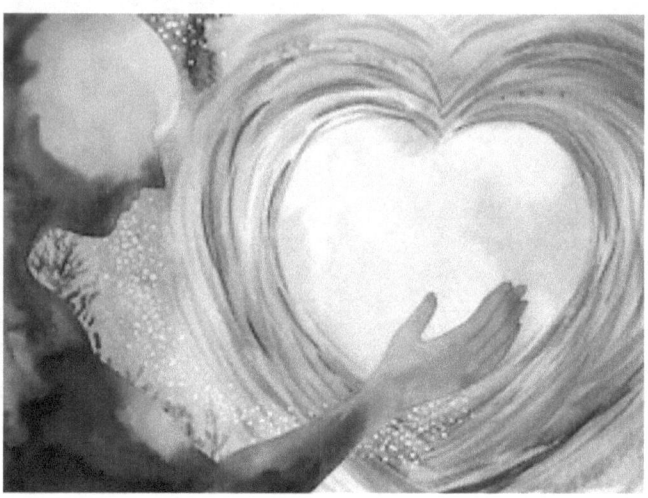

How to Choose a Chiropractor: The crazy thing about our profession is that a patient may walk into five different chiropractic clinics and experience five totally different methods. At one location, they want X-rays while others don't require it. Some may adjust by hand, others with tools. Some rub, heat, ice, shake and bake, while others use electrodes, creams and lotions. You may learn about a product line for improved nutrition, pumps, braces, shoes, etc., zero conformity within our great profession. You see, the chiropractor has learned so much about our natural healing capabilities, that all of these tools can aid in pointing you toward the direction of wellness. But where we get lost is failing to educate the patient on subluxation and the removal thereof. So let's simplify this message and teach the public about our great profession using the left and right analogy. On the far left is the straight "hole in one" (HIO) chiropractor, who only adjusts the atlas bone, C1. And as we progress from straight to mixer, slow shift from left to right, we will next have the chiropractors who adjust the whole spine. A principled chiropractor will always adjust the spine!

Further toward the mixer, we see the spine and extremity adjuster. As we continue our right shuffle we now have added the docs who use ice and heat. As we move from straight to even more of a mixer, we see the spinal adjuster, extremity adjuster, ice, heat, stretches, and traction. As we continue mixing possibly the work-out rehab doctor, the farther we travel toward the opposite end of the HIO doctor we may even run into a chiropractor who will do so much physical therapy and ignores the spine, in fact he does everything for the patient except remove subluxation, and that I have a problem with! Don't dilute the message. We chiropractors do something very unique and special. Anyone can rub a muscle and hook up electrodes, but to correct VSC is magnificent, therefore don't shortchange the blessing. I use to be a mixer when I got out of school. I always adjusted the spine but included many other therapies on the patient that upon leaving, they had no idea what it was that got them feeling better. Was it the ice, massage, traction, stretching, adjustment, decompression? When I focused on adjustments only, the patient got better and knew it was 100 percent related to the adjustment. I removed the confusion. Sure I incorporated posture correction techniques or stretch as homework, challenged them to make nutritional changes and increased their exercise rituals, etc. I've been able to focus on spinal care, my specialty, while treating more people.

The educated patient pays, stays, refers, and gets well, while continuing to thrive. I teach patients about subluxation on every visit and as soon as they walk out my door they forget it all! Why? This is the hard part about my profession, and it's very frustrating for chiropractors. Patients see the daily billion dollars of drug advertisement money that is spent by "Big Pharma" and have successfully managed to brainwash the public. This book will serve as a go-to educational guide, allowing the chiropractor to focus on the healing adjustment and not have to constantly teach. The patients should become very discerning towards spinal care via the education learned from this book and therefore start to seek out chiropractors everywhere. Patients should as a result of proper education via this book, flood to the chiropractors worldwide, blessing these public healers and the community as a whole as we witness an elevated level of health and wellness throughout the lands.

Polarized opinion: So many chiropractors have healed hundreds of thousands of people while others have caused the patient to hurt worse after care and tainted that individual from ever seeking chiropractic care again. Please try another chiropractor, and don't give up! Sometimes pain is inevitable prior to wellness making its appearance. It takes time for symptoms to show up, even more time for disease, so please be patient and stay adjusted. Healing may take a visit, a week, a month or even a season or two. Never give up when it comes to your health. Demand the best and remain consistent with your care. We chiropractors are a diverse bunch, change doctors if you are stuck in a wellness plateau.

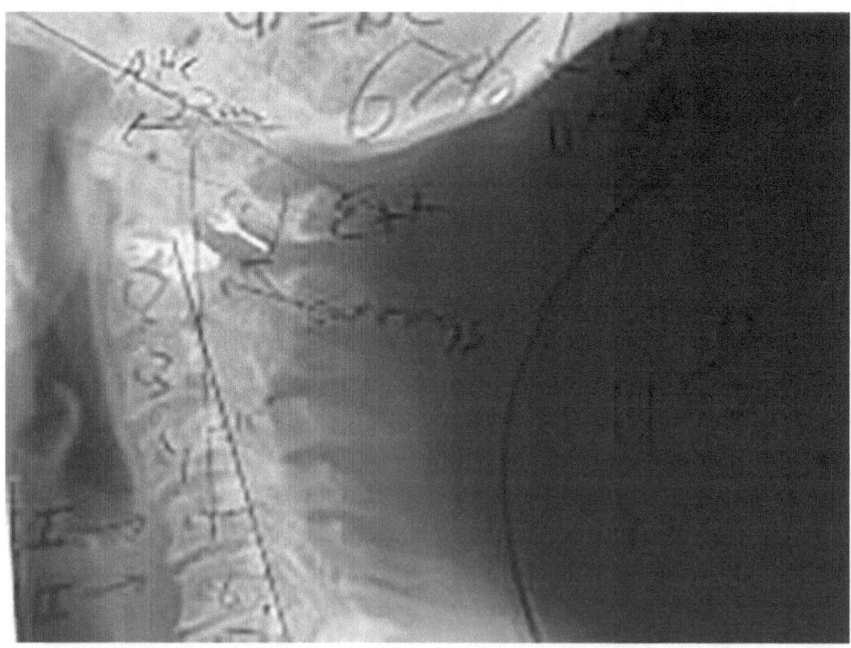

Should I have an x-ray taken (if necessary)? I believe that X-rays give you a starting blueprint of what the frame and joints look like, rule out pathology and are very helpful in cases where the patient is age forty or above. Radiology helps with case studies where a huge impact took place and trauma or pathology is expected. At age forty, we start to see degenerative changes as evidence on these films, bone thinning, X-ray variants as they pertain to the spine and so forth. So I believe the X-ray information is very useful in the correction process and to ensure accurate care. To see is to know, and not to see is to guess and I don't like to guess when it comes to my patient's health. Some chiropractors, like me, specialize in reduction of disc bulges, disc herniation, disc tears, and arthritis reversal, etc. which can be very painful for the patient, but if they continue with chiropractic care, wellness results start to show up within 2 months or less.

If the patient is under the age of 40 it's a case by case doctor's decision if X-rays are needed or not, based on symptoms, trauma, and severity of conditions, etc.

Chiropractic is always non-force, gentle and accurate. No twisting ever or violent slamming moves with multiple popping sounds. The adjustment is precision care with the isolation of one segment being adjusted at a time. The adjustment is always given to the locked or fixated joint, a.k.a. subluxation. How will the doctor find the proper locked joint to correct, by motion palpating each spinal segment! The joints that are in their proper position will not be tender to the touch and have a spongy end motion feel to them; they will wiggle when pushed on. The locked, fixated, VSC joint is very tender to the touch and feels more like the brick wall, no joint play when pushed upon. The chiropractor will use orthopedic test and possible X-rays to confirm his diagnosis. Patient also grimaces in pain when the locked joint is touched, bingo; you are on the correct segment that needs to be corrected back into its proper position, a.k.a. adjusted.

The doctor uses a short lever and high speed adjustment by hand with low force and corrects this VSC. The doctor should teach you about spinal care, and offer diet and exercise tips to help you reach optimal wellness faster, this can be done at home through email, or if time permits, during the office visit. Many chiropractic doctors have weekly or monthly patient workshops to educate the public, take some of your friends and loved ones to them, the very life you save may be theirs.

First—"Spend all the time necessary to carefully and precisely find and correct a patient's problem. Do not be in a hurry. Check and recheck your x-ray, your palpation, instrumentation, motion palpation, and visualization."
Second—"Remember that Chiropractic always works. When it does not seem to, examine your application, but do not question the principle."
Third—"Be prepared when demand for Chiropractic care increases. Study the spinal column and the nervous system every chance you get."
"Our future will be our results."
Dr. Clarence S. Gonstead

If you are getting B-Z at the chiropractic office but not an "Adjustment", change doctors, subluxations must be removed for optimal health and wellness.
(Jeff Trigo, DC)

References: Many resources are available in today's market because the presence of social media and the sorts thereof. People are using their smart phones to find a chiropractor near them and if you are not on the search engines you are missing out. I love when patients are thankful that they are living well, absence of their original chief complaint / symptom; That presents an opportunity to remind them that God does the healing and that the chiropractor removes the interference. I don't stop there; I let them also know that the best way to thank me is by referring a loved one who may also be suffering and is clueless that a locked spinal joint is the cause, and to include their happy reviews on various sites (Google, Yelp, Facebook, etc.) These 5 star reviews that the patients give you last forever! Remember some reviews may be false and/or written up by a non-patient, other health care competition, etc., but in general they can be useful. All reviews should be acknowledged and thanked in return.

How to Pick a Mate: Why is love so complicated? Allow me to suggest a few helpful tips from a man who has already made all the mistakes and if you can learn from my mistakes you can save yourself a few broken hearts. Don't give your heart away so easy thus preserve and protect it. God cherishes you and doesn't want you to share this love with a bunch of other people. We were designed to fall in love and have one mate. Where we are weak the mate is strong and vice versa. Where one may have great logic, know-how capabilities, and have problem solving skills, the other partner may possess feelings, emotions, empathy and intuition that must not be ignored. We complete each other. When united the two different people become one flesh. Everything about the mate matters more than self. Selfless never ending love that never fails! Men repent from sin, find joy in living a righteous life and keep your relationship solid with our Heavenly Father, the Son and the Holy Spirit; do this for eternity! Be the leader in the home reflecting Christ like love towards your wife always. Sacrifice your life for her while preserving her purity. Supply her a safe, secure, loving and warm environment for her to live in. Hide nothing and be transparent in all areas of your life with her. Read the Word with her daily and start off each day knowing that this is a new day that you get to prove to her how much you love her; love never fails! Wives, submit to your husbands, this pleases the Lord, so do it for God. Respect your man and remember you are his equal not above or below him in anyway. Cling to his side for life, be supportive, encouraging while also living a transparent life. Marriage is two sinners that unite and become one flesh with the privilege of extending forgiveness and grace towards each other often. Forgive for the rest of your life, this is Christ like. So before you go falling in love and giving away your heart please consider these important facts and traits about a mate:

- Religious background can make or break a relationship. If you have similar beliefs then you may be able to move mountains together; if not, then it's fuel for tearing you two apart. Same faith matters because it's the foundation for everything in the marriage.
- Financial goals must be in alignment. Clear and precise goals that allow for a budget to be in place. Timetable for

achieving specific goals spelled out on a calendar. If one person is busy trying to pay the house payment while the other is off spending money every day on useless trinkets, then this is a receipt for disaster.

- Child raising goals. You must both be in agreement on how many kids you wish to have, the type of discipline you will incorporate into the household. Do you both agree on the anti-vaccination protocol or do you believe in injectable toxins? At what age they will receive their first cell phone, get their ears pierced, start to drive or date, etc. Do you want your kids to go to college and if so, you need to start saving at birth.

- Political views. If one loves Hillary Clinton while the other supports Donald Trump, well talk about a divided home. Good luck having an intimate relationship with your mate.

- Miscellaneous goals. Does one like to travel while the other doesn't? Does the type of car you drive matter? Is there a neat freak in the house living with an unorganized mess of a person? Are you a pet person while the other prefers other people's pets? All of these issues matter.

- I believe the best relationships start out as awesome friendships, not lust. A friendship that grew into love that morphed into marriage.

- Expectations in regards to sex and how often, etc. Happy wife happy life. The man and woman both need affection and want to be pursued and appreciated. Cheating is the number one cause of divorce! Don't do it. It's stupid and not worth it. Remain faithful or be subdivided and torn apart as divorce lawyers cash in on the big profits of divorce. Learn about the 5 love languages and communicate to your partner which love language best describes your needs.

- Describe 50 traits about a mate that you seek so God can deliver this person to you. Some of these traits can be about looks, but very few like hair and eye color, body type, etc. Mostly describe the person in great detail; the mate likes to do this for fun, the personality, hobbies, how that person treats you, family values, background, education, the more details the better. Describe mates temperament, is she or he forgiving, confident, successful, organized, etc. If the person smokes or not, tattoos, body piercings, etc. When this person comes along there is no mistake this time. This must be on paper and prayed about, you will attract it as it is written.

"Likewise you younger people, submit yourselves to your elders. Yes, all of you be submissive to one another, and be clothed with humility, for "God resists the proud, but gives grace to the humble." Therefore humble yourselves under the mighty hand of God, that He may exalt you in due time, casting all you care upon Him, for He cares for you. Be sober; be vigilant; because your adversary the devil walks about like a roaring lion, seeking whom he may devour. Resist him, steadfast in the faith, knowing that the same sufferings are experienced by your brotherhood in the world." (1 Peter 5:5–9)

Heaven or Hell: It is God's wish that no one would perish but come to the saving knowledge of the free gift of grace that exists in accepting Jesus as your Lord and Savior. By faith we are saved not by works, so no one gets to boast, our works don't get us to heaven, but by faith alone. With great faith comes works out of pure loving service. Nothing should ever be done with "self-minded intent" but in service for "God-minded intent." JOY (Jesus, Others, You), and in that order.

Every year, for approximately 13 years, I taught chiropractic technique at the Texas Chiropractic College (TCC), and while in TX for eighteen days teaching the Japan Chiropractic Association, during a break at the local coffee shop, I heard a man talking to many different people over a period of several days. This Bible belt state takes their freedom of religious choice and Christianity seriously.

PTL—praise the Lord! I got to meet this retired dentist named Randy and we became great friends and I always looked forward to meeting with him the following year. After my observations of

Randy's technique, I too learned a simple way to ask people about their faith. The answer to my question would provide me with a quick understanding of the participants Bible knowledge and faith. It is a very effective method of communicating with simplicity and straight to the point. Are you ready to learn the question because the answer will follow?

Q: If you died and went to Heaven and God asks you why should I let you in, what would you say? He would let them speak and talk all they wanted. After all, Randy was retired hanging out at a coffee shop. When they were all done speaking he would either congratulate them on knowing the correct answer, assured in their salvation; or ask them if they would like to know what the Bible says?

A: Jesus is the first word that should come out of their mouths. Faith in Jesus that He came, He died, and He was raised from the dead on that third day. At the pearly gates point to Jesus and say, I know Him, He has me on His guest list in His Lambs Book of Life. I have been born again! Jesus is the truth and the only way, amen.

I have heard many wrong answers, because I am good person. I try not to sin. I'm a good dad, mom, husband, or wife. I go to church every Sunday, etc., all of these are works. Only by faith we are saved! If you are a believer, you're Heaven bound if not, I'm sorry but there is only "ONE WAY", and it's JESUS.

"For God so loved the world that He gave His only begotten Son, that whoever believes in Him should not perish but have ever lasting life." (John 3:16)

So to not believe is still making a choice and unfortunately if you were to die, you cannot go to heaven. Jesus is the way the truth and the life. No one is perfect, we need a Savior and salvation is easy. You must believe that He came, He died and He rose again. God's gift to the world was His Son, He seals us with the Holy Spirt as a reminder that God is always with us till the very end.

"Thou art worthy, O Lord, to receive glory and honour and power: for thou hast created all things, and for thy pleasure they are and were created." (Revelations 4:11)

Healthcare or Sick care: Take care of you master system and joint motion by receiving regular chiropractic care and you will love the results. Keep popping pills and scheduling procedure after procedure, test after test; surgeries and the sorts thereof, you will have a sickness story and continue living life as a victim with some disease label which I think is totally absolutely ludicrous. There is another way that is scientific and proven. This method works. Healing takes time and as long as you are doing everything you can daily to live a healthy lifestyle, the wellness results are eminent. Just don't make the common mistake that many do by ignoring your spine. The medical field in general will ignore subluxation and therefore mostly never refer you to a chiropractor, so you must take back control of your own wellness destiny by choosing for yourself the best path. If a simple adjustment or a small series of adjustments will correct the underlying problem, wouldn't that be a better and a safer choice versus a pill popping pain management regimen that masks cause, while ignoring causation and definitely brings about adverse side effects? Remember this statement:

"Everybody has subluxations, therefore every spine matters." (Jeff Trigo, DC)

www.TrigoChiropractic.com

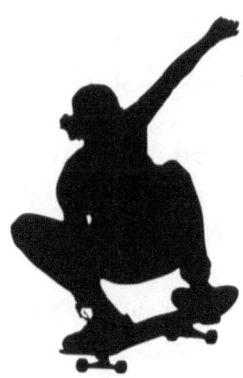

Whether or not you believe me doesn't change the fact that you have a spine that is locked or will become locked in at least one spinal location or more. Choose to fix VSC with regularity and watch symptoms disappear like a puddle on a hot day. Train your body, eat the rainbow of life and keep your eyes on Heavenly things.

"Live long and prosper." (Spock, Leonard Nimoy)

Positive or Negative: Nobody wants to be around a negative person that is always dumping their problems on others while, blame shifting and ignoring good advice. Don't play the part of a victim, which is always telling your stories of woes. Heaping them upon un-expectant ears when asked how are you today? Celebrate your victories and be glad in them. Count your blessings and keep your mind on contentment while putting together a plan of success to overcome. Have a close group of godly friends nearby that you can confide in and they will pray for you. Then leave those woes at the cross. Trust in Him who loves you to deliver you, mold you, refine you, and make you better for His purpose and kingdom expansion. Regardless of today's troubles, these will pass as they refine you. Remember that you're still a beloved royal member in God's family, live like it, because you are His royal priesthood. Enjoy each day 100 percent. We never know when our last day will arrive, so love, laugh, witness, serve and tell others to buy this book, if it has helped you. I guarantee it will also help others.

Be the example you want to see in the world: Happiness with great contentment can be contagious. We sometimes do not see the bigger purpose when we are in various trials, but this has happened before, and there is nothing new under the sun. Remember while Jonah was in the belly of the whale, he was praying for that second chance and God was moving behind the scenes just like that great fish was moving and swimming toward the land that God commanded him to go to. Pray continuously and the squeaky wheel gets the oil. God loves to answer our prayers if it will bring Christ the glory and is in Gods loving nature. Most of all be patient, God timing is better than our timing. Remain faithful and true to yourself, be the best version of you that you can possible be and enjoy every breath you get on this planet. Live in the present, forgive your past, because Jesus took away those sins and made you perfect in His redemption, and goal set for the future. Celebrate your achieved goals with your loved ones and then set new outrageous ones.

Jesus said "These things I have spoken unto you, that in me ye might have peace. In the world ye shall have tribulations: but be of good cheer; I have overcome the world." (John 16:33)

Are you doing as much as you can for the people around you? How can you leave the world a better place than you found it? I have never seen a moving truck following a hearse, you can't take all your stuff with you so help others while you can. Donate time and "stuff" to your loved ones while you are still alive, they won't be able to fight over it when you're gone!

"Once you make the choice to possess a good attitude, the work really begins. Now comes a life of continual deciding to grow and maintaining the right outlook. Attitudes have a tendency to revert back to their original patterns if not carefully guarded and cultivated." (John C. Maxwell)

It takes more muscles to frown versus muscles needed to smile, so enjoy as many moments as you can and smile often, because people will notice. Share your life knowledge and pour into others. What you do is of greater importance than what you say so if you want to have a positive impact to those around you then be the example and lead by example and when necessary you can also use your words. We all have a limitless potential, but seldom do people try to reach for the stars. Remember we can do anything just not everything, surround yourself with an awesome team of overachievers and allow them to feel important, this will have a great outcome on the results you are trying to achieve. Always remember that the proper attitude you display toward anything will dictate performance.

BAG: Choose to pursue and accomplish your Big Audacious Goals a.k.a. "BAG." It's an amazing feeling that happens when you remove all obstacles, knocking down all the walls of resistance and celebrating your accomplishments. Go for it and never look back.

Big Challenge: Tame your tongue by guarding your speech, keeping it sweet and loving in all you do. Belief determines behavior and attitude reflects leadership. Our very lips praise our Father, while cursing our brother and this should not be so. We don't need more clowns or jokesters in this world, we need more people who will share the redemption story and represent Him well as we set the example and live this life for Him, always with eternity in mind.

> **"My lips will not speak wickedness, Nor my tongue utter deceit." (Job 27:4)**

Create daily gem moments that will leave embedded positive memories in your mind, go deep into your communion with God and then create meaningful relationships that last with Christ as the Cornerstone.

Don't hesitate to tell others about this book, because if we can make this information go viral and the words fall upon ears that hear, eyes that see and hearts that are open, then we can really make a huge change together, one soul, one spine and one mind at a time, in Jesus name, Amen.

The Bible wasn't only written for our information or even our inspiration, but for our transformation, so don't be conformed but transformed. Stay "Heavenly Minded" folks. Righteousness is the emptying of self and becoming more like Jesus and the fullness of His Spirit in us that makes us righteous.

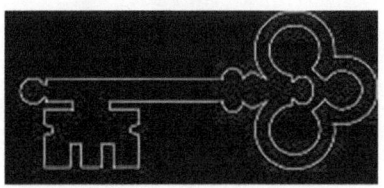

"For as he thinks within himself, so he is." Proverbs 23:7

May the light of the Holy Spirit shine within your heart because with Jesus, your life becomes more meaningful and exciting. This knowledge of the King gives us a living hope in every situation and in every environment. Life is not just better with Jesus, It's the best with Jesus, body, soul and spirit. With man, it is impossible to please God, however a good start would be kneeling more often in prayer. Praise Him daily, confess your sins on a regular basis, and show gratitude for your many blessings, while offering prayer on the behalf of others. Remember the acronym for this prayer style; ACTS. His unending grace and love will never fail us! We are members in His Holy family.

"For by grace you have been saved through faith, and that not of yourselves; it is the gift of God." Ephesians 2:8 NKJV

Choosing to stay motivated while giving 100% effort to the day will keep your mind busy and protect you from harming yourself and others. Integrity is doing what's right even when no one is looking this develops character. Stay focused so you can achieve your goals. Remember that every choice has consequences so think it well through before you decide what to do. Develop routines!

A poem from a dear friend and faithful
servant of Calvary Chapel Beachside:

Long Ago
Across The Sea
Born Divine
Set Man Free
Inside A Manger
Beneath A Star
3 Wise Strangers
Came Afar
Bearing Gifts
Befit A King
The Heavens Shift
As Angels Sing
Glory Glory
Men Of Earth
For Comes Today
A Virgin's Birth
Born Of God
No Sin Inside
He Came For All
So None Would Die

So Let Us Sing
Songs Of Praise
His Only Son
Who Came To Save
Rejoice My Friends
He's Still Alive
We're Born Again
He Lives Inside
Rejoice In Spirit
Heavens Above
For In Our Hearts
We Have His Love
Rejoice With Friends
With Family
Rejoice In Jesus
Who Set You Free
By Kevin Kown

CHAPTER 16

Q&A with the Patients

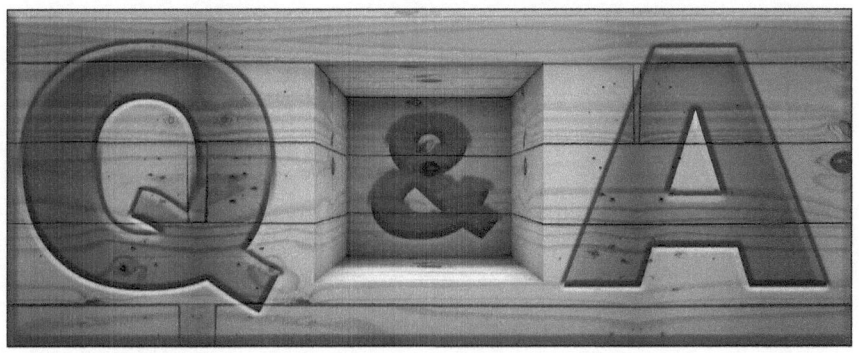

Q: How come it hurts in the morning when I wake up and through-out the day as I start moving around, it starts to feel a little better?

A: We have a sealed "hydraulic-like" cerebral spinal fluid pumping system that moves in and throughout our spinal column and joints. This fluid gets its high oxygen content through ventricles located in the spaces between brain lobes and then travels down the spine. Subluxation inhibits the free flow of spinal fluid in and out of the disc and joint space therefore upon waking the patient with subluxation feels dehydrated sore and starving for lubrication. Even though the joints are locked, the joint has micro-movement that will cause limited lubrication thus eas-ing some of the tension only to return the next day upon waking. This is a common example of the expression of a classic subluxation.

Q: I hear that chiropractic can be addicting and once you start chiropractic care you will always need to go to the chiropractor?

A: The truth is that chiropractic care is so effective for fixing subluxation that when life produces these subluxations, the only way to get rid of them is by a chiropractic adjustment. It's very addicting to feel good and chiropractic adjustments restore joint motion and nervous system function so fast and affordably that patients choose to stay adjusted for maximum long term wellness.

Q: What's the best position to sleep in doc?

A: We spend 1/3 of our life sleeping, so invest in a good firm bed that is flippable and rotatable. The position we sleep in matters. Bad sleeping habits can really misalign your spine while other positions are more natural and can reinforce stability. I prefer side posture with a support pillow between the knees and a large pillow that supports the head in a neutral position. This position will have your head level and ears over the center of the shoulders. If the pillow is too large or small when sleeping in side posture, the cervical spine will be laterally flexed and neck pressure will exist. This can cause misalignments, numbness in upper limbs or increased disc pressure even tears of the disc fibers.

If you lay on your back please use a thin pillow with arch support to help restore the natural spinal curves. Stomach sleeping must be avoided, this causes the neck to over rotate, causing upper cervical brain stem pressure which I have found to be very prevalent in today's day and age. 90 percent of all my patients have upper cervical pressure and text neck, always looking down, it is pandemic!

Q: How much schooling does it take to become a chiropractor?

A: The values below represent class hours.

Chiropractic	Course	Medicine
540	Anatomy	508
240	Physiology	326
360	Pathology	401
165	Chemistry	325
120	Microbiology	114
630	Diagnosis	324
320	Neurology	112
360	X-Ray	148
60	Psychiatry	144
60	Obstetrics	148
210	Orthopedics	156
3065	**Total**	**Hours** **2706**

Other Required Subjects
Spinal Adjustments Pharmacology
Nutrition Immunology
Advance Radiology General Surgery

4485   **4248**

Q: At what age should one begin to see the chiropractor for spinal health?

A: The birthing process is usually very traumatic, both for the baby and the mother. Fact is, most subluxations begin at birth and are the cause for colic symptoms in babies (always crying—they're in pain), SIDS (sudden infant death syndrome), ear infections, asymmetrical range of motion with neck turning, digestive disorders and so much more. I always tell my patients:

"Stay Adjusted from the Womb to the Tomb." (Jeff Trigo, DC)

Q: Is chiropractic care safe for pregnant patients?

A: Absolutely! This drug free approach to healing is especially useful during pregnancy. In fact many chiropractors take extra courses on how to correct breach babies, and have regularly obtained outstanding results in getting the baby into the proper position for the birthing process. Chiropractic will help the spine, pelvis and other related structures remain in proper balance, free of subluxation and maintaining proper joint movement and nerve supply for mother during this joyful time. Chiropractic adjustments ensure that mom doesn't have to be suffering heartburn, sciatic, vomiting (first trimester), loss of pregnancy and other common conditions such as back pain that affects third trimester expecting mothers to be. During pregnancy, usually no X-rays are taken; no vibration therapy given that may shake the baby. No ultra-sound that may penetrate too deep, no aggressive drop tables are used, etc. In postpartum care (after birth), women return for spinal realignments to reduce whatever birthing trauma took place during birth, thus helping the mother recover faster and safer. This is a drug free natural approach to health which will preserve the integrity of the breast milk from which the baby should feed on for the first year of life.

Q: If I have osteoporosis (bone thinning) is it safe to get adjusted?

A: When a person turns forty hormonal changes occur in which we stop putting mineral deposits into bone and start withdrawing from them. Osteoporosis is a condition in which mineral deposits get pulled out of the bone and put into the blood stream. A diet that is high in minerals can avoid this problem; where the density can be depleted and subjected to pathological fractures. If the bones have already undergone density depletion one fact still remains, it affects the vertebral body of the vertebra only and the chiropractor will not ever come into contact with this area as adjustments are being given. The chiropractor adjusts the vertebra in an area that is not affected by bone thinning. This area is the spinous process, or the transverse process or even the mammillary process. Bone thinning will never affect these regions and therefore when a chiropractor gently pushes the bone forward off the nerve, it's 100 percent safe and therapeutical.

Bending forward while lifting heavy objects puts increased pressure on the body of the vertebra and this is what causes pathological fractures. Lift with your legs not with your back.

Q: How long does it take to correct vertebral subluxation, because every time I get adjusted it just eventually pops out again doc?

A: Similar to the time it which it takes to correct the alignment of the teeth; 2 years of braces and 1 year of a retainer, the spine also has a corrective protocol. The spinal corrective process is much more difficult because we are constantly in motion and bad postural habits need to also be corrected for the adjustments to hold longer. Another factor that one must take into account is the amount of damage and/or degeneration that has crept into the spinal segments due to long term subluxation. The sooner care begins the easier it is for the spinal ligaments to hold the bone into its new position. It takes approximately 40 adjustments to make a permanent change visible on X-ray. Pressure over time creates the change. If a person is only getting once a week adjustments, I found that within 1 to 1.5 years the upper neck region, a.k.a. brain stem, is corrected and holding from week to week. This time represents a maximum time and I've seen it correct much sooner. However when a motivated patient comes twice a week, I've seen great correction obtained within 3-4 months. The phase 2 degenerated spinal joint can take 2-4 years to correct and the phase 3 degenerated spinal joint can take 3-5 years to correct. I have before and after X-ray films where the phase 3 disc degeneration (bone on bone) is now hydrated and appears to have a large space between the vertebras. Stenosis was resolved and the patient feels wonderful. The spurs don't go away but they are not the problem, it's the pinched nerve and locked joint that is the problem. Once you remove that impingement and unlock the joint, function returns and the spurs no longer need to grow. The spurs are growing to fuse an unstable joint. The body does this to preserve and protect what little nerve function is left. However, when the stability is returned to the joint, the fusion process ceases. After correction and stability is obtained (defined by a spine that can hold for 2 weeks), then the patient is put on maintenance care at a frequency of every 2 weeks unless their job or hobbies are extreme then I suggest a frequency of once a week as my best recommendation.

Q: After I got adjusted I slept so well and an extra couple hours too, do you think the adjustment had anything to do with it doc?

A: One thing for sure is that plenty of healing takes place while you are asleep. If your adjustment has allowed you to sleep like a baby again, that awesome, it's a welcomed benefit of turning the body's power back on. Brain stem pressure is the major cause of insomnia and fixing the alignment of C1 is the first step to getting your wellness back. Great sleep is an important factor that must be restored ASAP. It will lower stress and help to regulate normal blood pressure.

> **"So many people spend their health gaining wealth, and then have to spend their wealth to regain their health." (A. J. Reb Materi)**

Q: Is an adjustment the only thing that the chiropractor does during the office visit?

A: The Doctor of Chiropractic has a great amount of tools in his bag of tricks that can be used on various different visits. Performing orthopedic tests to determine diagnosis of soft tissue injuries. Radiographic studies are often taken to rule out pathology, diagnose misalignments; also muscle testing is available to help determine areas of nerve compromise. The chiropractor is well trained in physical therapy and rehabilitation techniques. Nutritional changes can also be implemented as needed to aid in healing. Other modalities include: disc decompression, foot levelers, postural corrective exercise and stretches. With this great wellness knowledge, the chiropractor will know how and when to treat you, when to refer you out, as appropriate and to whom, and even when to co-manage by using other health care practitioners in conjunction with spinal corrective adjusting techniques that best suit your spinal needs.

Changing your perspective on the healing process will help you to persevere and obtain the true wellness that you desire. Just know that subluxations will happen no matter what you do to prevent them, therefore stay adjusted and live a life without fear. Push yourself and never compromise your integrity.

Q: Is chiropractic effective in treating arthritis?

A: So many different types of arthritis respond well to the welcomed return of joint motion. In fact all untreated subluxation have a destiny called arthritis therefore if we introduce motion into the spine the lubrication process returns thus aiding and even reversing this degenerative inflammatory process.

"One of the best aspect of health care reform is to start emphasizing prevention." (Anne Wojcicki)

Q: I have had spinal fusion surgery, can I still see a chiropractor?

A: Once the vertebral joint has undergone spinal fusion, that joint is now locked into its surgical position. Often times screws are used to anchor the bone into a permanent position. Chiropractic will absolutely be beneficial for the regions above and below the surgical site. Research shows that 95 percent of all surgical procedures on the spine have a return in the original symptoms by the fifth year. It is my hope that any and all patients would try up to 4 different chiropractors before undergoing spinal surgery. Surgery should always be a last resort due to the invasiveness when compared to a gentle chiropractic corrective adjustment.

Q: Should I go to the chiropractic doctor before the medical doctor or the MD before the DC?

A: Chiropractors are the neuro-muscular-skeletal specialist. If you are experiencing those types of symptoms then chiropractic is best. I like to give analogies for better understanding and public education, so I will put it like this, chiropractic is like the carpenter and the medical doctor is like the fire department. If your house is on fire (heart attack, busted colon and toxins are spilling into your body, brain tumor, etc.) then you need the fire department to save the building with their axes, hammers and hoses, a.k.a. surgical intervention. If you have maintenance or remodeling needs it will look pretty funny if the fire department shows up with their axes and hose. In other words you will now need the finish carpenter to do the necessary upkeep to prevent the body's crisis (fire) from happening. Chronic pain syndromes acute pain and various other conditions like numbness, etc. should first be under chiropractic care. Let the chiropractor be the doctor who will refer you out if the condition is out of the scope of this great profession. Most conditions resolve with chiropractic and with prevention many conditions can be avoided.

Q: When I turn my head left and right it feels like there is sandpaper grinding in my neck, do you know what that is doc?

A: When a subluxation has been present for any length of time, our normal 45 degree neck curve is usually compromised thus anterior head carriage (AHC) is commonly found upon examination. This neck curve acts like a shock absorber for the weight of the head which is approximately 12-15 pounds. For every 1 inch in AHC, the weight of the head doubles on the disc. This increase in disc load contributes to the fluid being squeezed out of the disc. This is comparative to squeezing a sponge and having the water ooze out. This loss of water content in a disc gives us a sandpaper grinding sensation because lubrication is compromised. Dried out discs feel like sandpaper granules upon rotation, this is called crepitus. A wonderful benefit of receiving chiropractic care is that this usually goes away with proper curve restoration and the welcomed return of normal joint motion.

Q: Should I use ice or heat on this doc?

A: The rule is as follows, new injury first 48 hours (acute) it's best to ice. RICE—rest, ice, compress, elevate. When I say ice that means five to eight minutes with a very thin barrier like a T-shirt or paper towel. Once you put the ice on yourself you will experience 4 stages: Cold, ache, burning, numbness. This process only takes 5-8 minutes. I suggest an am, noon and pm routine for the first 2 days of an injury. After 48 hours (chronic) it's best to start using moist heat. This is important, because a heating pad that plugs into the wall is not moist heat. A wet towel out of the microwave or hot water, bath, spa, shower are all moist heat. Dry heat is contraindicated in all neuro-muscular-skeletal conditions. Dry heat increases adhesions and scar tissue. Chronic injuries also respond well to contrast which is moist heat first, then ice, then moist heat again. This literally pumps open and closes the vessels and helps reduce swelling while increasing blood flow necessary for oxygen delivery for a faster healing process.

Q: When I look at pictures taken of me, it looks like my head is always tilted, what does that mean doc?

A: The great chiropractic coach C. J. Mertz, DC, said that "Posture is the window to the spine"! In other words, as the twig is bent so grows the tree. If you have a head tilt there is a 100 percent chance that you have upper neck subluxations and need an adjustment yesterday. Chiropractors specialize in the correction of subluxation while permanently improving your posture for maximum healthy benefits.

Q: I was told that I have one leg shorter than the other, was I born like this and is this causing my back pain?

A: Actually it's quite the opposite, when the pelvis and sacrum area is out of alignment, this common problem can create a long or short leg. The goal is to adjust the locked sacroiliac joint (SI joint) and create a level foundation in which the whole spine sits upon. We are born with very symmetrical extremity lengths, arms and legs; you were not born with that discrepancy. You most likely had a trauma. Life produces many traumatic falls thus dislodging the pelvic foundation and creating this unleveled leg length appearance.

**"Wisdom is not a product of schooling but
of the lifelong attempt to acquire it"
Albert Einstein**

Q: Do chiropractors just adjust the spine or can they adjust other areas of the body?

A: Besides spinal adjustment, chiropractors can also adjust fingers, wrist, elbows, shoulders, clavicles, toes, feet, ankles, knees, hips, sutures, jaws, and more.

Q: What will I feel after an adjustment, will it hurt?

A: People respond to chiropractic adjustments in their own unique way. One thing you have to remember is that healing takes time and the sooner the adjustment is given the better, because this action will minimize the damage that can infiltrate the affected areas. After an adjustment common reactions felt amongst mostly everybody include: A relaxed feeling, while knowing that the cause of your health ailments is being removed creating increased mental and physical satisfaction. You will notice a decrease in pain and other symptoms that you presented to the chiropractor originally with. Improved energy, balance and posture. Solid sleep with increase vigor and energy. The body can also pick and choose which symptom it wants to rid itself of first so stay patient and keep your spine adjusted so that the body can go through the healing process without hindrance while maximizing long term benefits.

Q: Why should I get adjusted if I'm feeling fine?

A: Most subluxations we don't even feel. It has been said that 90 percent of the nerve needs to be crushed before pain shows up, therefore it's important to stay regular with your care and not wait for symptoms. This is called taking health matters into your own hands by being proactive. You wouldn't wait for a cavity to show up before you start brushing your teeth, well the spine is actually more important than you teeth. Stay adjusted on a regular basis and experience true wellness not only absent of disease but thrive and live a life full of energy and vigor. Life flows from above, down, inside-out, these neuro-electrical impulses control the body's health from the brain to the tissue-cell and back to the brain.

"The wellness and prevention market will outgrow the health care market" Leroy Hood

Q: I was told that if I had a disc problem I have to get surgery or injections and to stay away from the chiropractor?

A: Chiropractors have many treatment methods when it comes to disc injuries. First off, all subluxations start the disc toward the path of degenerative pathology. Restoring joint motion is very important in the hydrating process. Disc decompression and traction will help to reabsorb the bulges and herniation. Lumbar rocking methods along with other adjunct therapies like Posture Pumps sold and made in Huntington Beach, have proven very successful in treating disc injuries. Pre and post MRIs have shown reduction and correction of large disc herniation, up to 10mm and more, post corrective chiropractic care which included the special disc work necessary to see such results. The goal is to create long term stability and health to the region and with disc injuries, slow and steady wins the race. Flexion must be avoided and even though disc tears are very painful, it usually takes about 2-4 weeks to successfully acquire at least 50 percent improvement in these painful conditions. Be patient and listen to what your chiropractor is asking you do at home. Ice helps to reduce the swelling and don't miss any appointments. I have had so many successful cases that responded great to chiropractic care, and I have had others who after one visit went the M.D. route, because they were impatient and wanted a quick fix. News flash, there is no quick fix and 95 percent of all low back surgeries get a return of original symptoms within the first 5 years or less. So don't lose trust in the process and healing takes time so don't give up. Ever!

"People who get regular care never show up with a disc tear." (Jeff Trigo, DC)

Q: Can I work out after an adjustment?

A: I often get asked this question and my common reply is "Live life without fear" Freddy Barge. In other words, if you stay adjusted you can enjoy activities like surfing, skateboarding, Jujitsu, etc. I would prefer one to have a well-adjusted spine upon any strenuous activity thus limiting injury. Do the things you enjoy doing, just take great care of your spine so your spine can take great care of you.

There is almost nothing you can't achieve. Identify what your talents and gifts are that God gave you and pursue your dreams and goals with zero hesitation. Live an extraordinary outrageous life and become successful beyond your wildest expectations. Believe it or not, God wants this for you, so never settle for mediocrity. Change can begin at any moment, now is a good time to start.

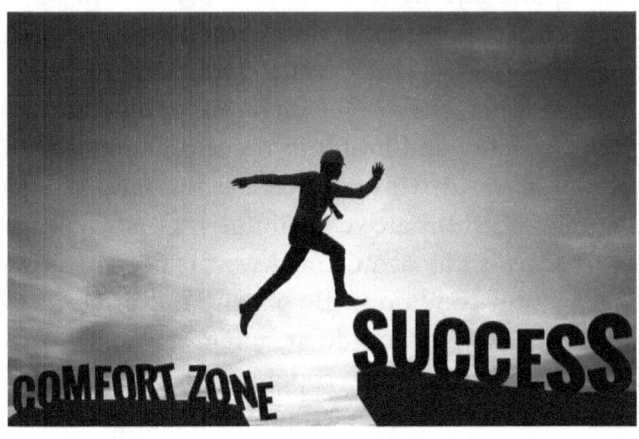

Humans were divinely designed to live here on earth. Mainstream media wants you to think that you were made incomplete and need their potions, lotions, shots, bolts and screws! Do not fall for their sickness ploys and big profit tactics. Learn to boost your immune system instead. A spine that is fine-tuned, a body well trained with proper supplementation, can easily kill virus, bacteria and so forth. Remember you have an Immune System! Chiropractic is a gift from Above, Down, from the Inside-Out, expect miracles! Read, learn and share this wisdom with as many people as possible. Take a picture holding this book and post it on your social media, I really need your help to make a difference. You can purchase this book via multiple platforms found on my web site www.TrigoChiropractic.com

CHAPTER 17

Final Exhortations

Celebrate the passing of each day with a gratitude for life, humility in mind and love in your heart. You were made perfect, absent of nothing. Keep your temple (body with Christ's Holy Spirit inside) pure, wholesome and simple. Practice forgiveness, live a life that is full of contentment and set outrageous goals. God wants the absolute best for you so don't stray away from Him. Become a prayer warrior and when you wake up in the morning, make the Devil think, oh darn, he or she is up again! Pray without ceasing, that's biblical. Sing praises to Him all day long and watch your life become full of JOY as you become more useful for His kingdom expansion. God wants you to live an abundant life so go for it, what are you waiting for?

**"Put away all pride so that you don't get
knocked off your high horse."
(Jeff Trigo, DC)**

If you don't know where you came from then how will you know where you are going and what's in store for you? People on earth fight over gold and that's asphalt in heaven. Money is very common, be extraordinary and seek things which are above. Heaven is above the earth and His ways are better than our ways. Trust in the Lord, He loves you and will dispense Angeles with flaming swords to protect you in times of need. Psalms 91:11. Remain faithful because

He loves you, therefore you can accomplish anything you put your heart toward as long as it brings glory to Christ, God's only begotten Son, and it is in the loving nature of God.

And the Lord said, "If you have faith as a mustard seed, you can say to this mulberry tree, 'Be pulled up by the roots, and be planted in the sea,' and it would obey you. Luke 17:6

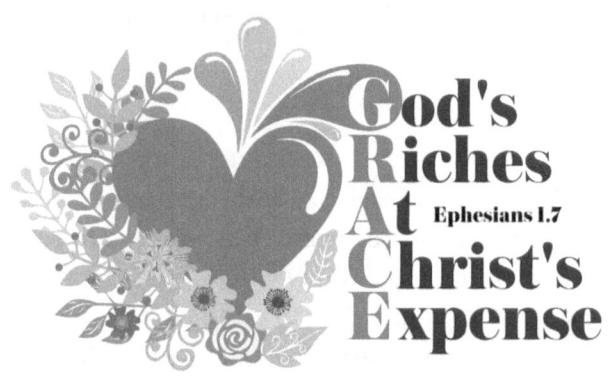

Health is earned and it's a proper lifestyle that obtains it. You will never find wellness in a medication pill bottle. Wealthy people on their death beds would spend their life fortunes to acquire more time on earth. With that in mind, don't hesitate, start your wellness plan now and don't wait for dis/ease. Make an appointment with a chiropractor nearby. I would love to help you with your spinal health by providing you tune ups to turn your power to heal back on. Chiropractors keep those pisiforms very polished. Don't let your MCP contact points rust away. Stay on purpose as we turn on function with that "tic" therefore allowing the inner healer, Innate Wisdom, to flourish as Universal Intelligence intended. Let action, the adjustment, be given without fear thus providing that source of healing power for all. Leave no spine behind; be bold with the message of chiropractic and its philosophy; brave telling the story to all. Finally be gentle, accurate, and precise. God bless you all that are gifted in the fine art of subluxation removal, you are truly being used by God to heal His people.

Join a gym yesterday and train 3-5 times a week. Eat real foods daily, every time you cheat with your diet you are sabotaging the great potential of the compound effect in your life. Guard your mind and only entertain what is positive and loving and do this by prayer and fasting if needed and keep yourself from evil wicked thoughts. Feed your mind with good loving thoughts and energy.

For the flesh lust against the Spirit, and the Spirit against the flesh; and these are contrary to one another, so that you do not do the things that you wish. Galatians 5:17

Surround yourself with likeminded people that have solid ethical values. Be the person that sets the example by doing, not all talk, but be a person of action. It is easy for a sinner to pull you down to their level so if you are a valued member in Gods Holy family, then soar with the eagles and don't sit with the turkeys!

"Let all bitterness, wrath, anger, clamor, and evil speaking be put away from you, with all malice. And be kind to one another, tenderhearted, forgiving one another, even as God in Christ forgave you."
Ephesians 4: 31-32

Where your heart is, so dwells your mind. For out of the mouth speaks the things of the heart. Let your communication be sweet, lifting up others and showing them that you care for them and that they are important to you.

Beware of these 3 hooks that the enemy uses as bait to hook you and tempt you:

1. Lust says, "I want it."
2. Entitlement says, "I deserve it."
3. Pride says, "I can handle it."

The devil is a very crafty enemy that has mastered the art of deception with his many lies, accusations, deceit and he enjoys playing the copycat / imposter. He will throw thoughts your way that include but not limited to: "not good enough", "unlovable", "having zero value or worth", "hopeless", "needing the next drug/ high to numb yourself" etc. Anger is his fuel and depression is his stepping stool. He will use greed to take your mind off God. While lust is his devouring monster that will consume you like a cancer as it grows inside of your mind leading to corruption and feeding the flesh instead of the Holy Spirit that dwells in the righteous individual. Don't bite the shiny fish lures that hook and kill. Be aware of his evil tactics so that you too can recognize them and run away like Joseph did when Potiphar's wife approached him in a sinful, lusting way.

Likewise you younger people, submit yourselves to your elders. Yes, all of you be submissive to one another, and be clothed with humility, for "God resists the proud, but gives grace to the humble." Therefore humble yourselves under the mighty hand of God, that He may exalt you in due time, casting all you care upon Him, for He cares for you. Be sober; be vigilant; because your adversary the devil walks about like a roaring lion, seeking whom he may devour. Resist him, steadfast in the faith, knowing that the same sufferings are experienced by your brotherhood in the world (1 Peter 5: 5–9).

The compound effect can always be in motion in our daily lives. Are these effects adding up to wellness or dis/ease? Poverty or riches? Amazing relationships or loneliness? Are they serving God in Heaven or the Devil and self? You get to decide which direction you are heading. You are the master of your own life so be accountable for your actions and success or failures. The key to your life depends on your daily actions. What you think, where you go, what captivates your thoughts, and how you will act are all under your direct control, that's good news! It's not good luck its God luck!

Break all your bad habits, embrace newer healthier ones and begin the exciting journey of the new and improved updated version of you. This new version would never go two weeks without a spinal adjustment that would just be preposterous! Your new mindset is one of gratitude, forgiveness and living in grace where hope abounds, and mental stability exists thereof. Stay active with regular hard physical exercise, you will never regret that sweat equity that you expended. Everything you consume is healthy because it really matters what you put in your mouth. This includes no more running to the pharmacy but allowing adequate time for natural healing to take place. Pharmacy is the last resort no longer the first! Wellness and preventative care is at the foremost part of your mind implemented into a daily action plan with measurable results. This next level of you really cares about others and put their needs before self. Always having the mindset of love, peace and patience. Remember to never sabotage the compound effect in any area of your life and or goals. That little extra push and your willpower to say on purpose really adds up over time. "Just Do It" Nike! It may take time for your loved ones to notice the change in you; a renewed person living by grace, with a positive passion for life. Just remember this, when people notice your joy and ask you what has changed? Your reply should include:

Christ in you, the hope of Glory. Colossians 1:27

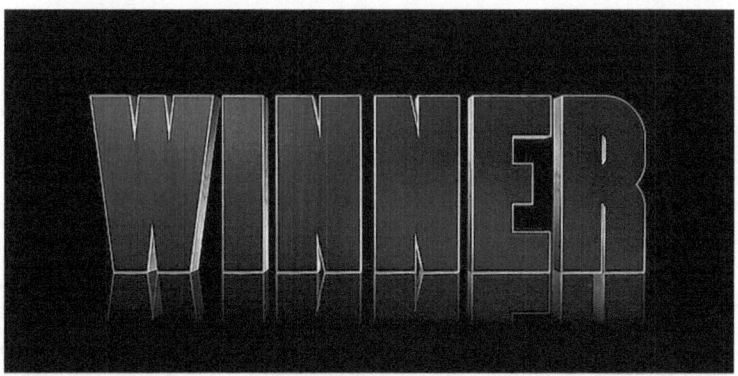

Goals should always include helping others to reach their highest potentials in all the areas of their life (salvation, relationships, health, finances, etc.). Serve more, love more and put others first more often. In doing so you will find out what kind of effects this will have upon your own life. Great JOY is obtained when others are put before self, Christ really gets to pour into you when you serve others.

Are you contemplating much, a giant at thought, deeply pondering and gazing yet actions are stagnant or dwarfed? You need to identify your goals and set sail; constantly "adjusting" your rudder while keeping your compass, aka actions, in "alignment" with your goals. This axiom takes on a higher significance when you realize who our identity is in Christ or LORD. For if He is for us, then who can be against us. We all die, it's how we live that matters!

Have you been neglecting your spine, by definition going longer than two weeks without an adjustment? If so then you definitely have a symptom story. Remember this, physical, emotional and chemical stressors can subluxated anyone! Heck even gravity can knock a spinal vertebra out. We must stop neglecting our spines. Teach them in their youth! Yell it from the roof tops, ignore spinal wellness no more! Get proactive and put away any trepidation you may be experiencing towards that corrective gentle adjustment; it actually feels great to remove VSC. You can have a wellness life or a sickness story. One takes education and action while the other ignorance and neglect, it's your choice.

**Success is defined by doing what you
love, and loving what you do.
Not by any balance sheets! Jeff Trigo, D.C.**

The hardest part of wellness is not the healing, the body is great at that when the nerve interference is removed. It's teaching the patient how spinal locks contribute to their diminished health, the spinal adjustment commitment needed, and the follow-through skills which lack. I wish to hear more of the people's wellness story, do you have one, and is it written on paper, has it been established?

"Control your own destiny or someone else will." Jack Welsh

Natural healing is scientific and powerful. Remember that God doesn't make junk! Always try the non-invasive natural approach to healing first not last. Change is possible and it can happen one spine at a time and every spine matters. Please help me to get this book out to the four corners of the earth by recommending it to all of your loved ones ASAP. Together we can increase health while removing the cause of dis/ease, stop unnecessary surgeries and pill dispensing while saving souls by spreading the good news:

Jesus came, He died, He rose again, and we are a forgiven people in Him our Lord and Savior. Please say this prayer today so that in case your last day comes you will know that you have a valid passport to heaven: Father God in Heaven, I'm a sinner and I need a Savior! You sent your Son into the world to die in my place, and it's by faith in the finished work of Jesus Christ on the cross that I am forgiven and welcomed into your kingdom. I welcome you Jesus to become the Lord of my life as I follow you all the rest of my days here on earth. Father God in Heaven thank you for your awesome plan of redemption that was made possible in the death and resurrection of Jesus Christ my Lord and Savior, in Jesus name I pray Amen.

(For this reason I bow my knees to the Father of our Lord Jesus Christ, From whom the whole family in heaven and earth is named, that He would grant you, according to the riches of His glory, to be strengthened with might through His Spirit in the inner man, that Christ may dwell in your hearts through faith; that you, being rooted and grounded in love, may be able to comprehend with all the saints what is the width and length and depth and height—to know the love of Christ which passes knowledge; that you may be filled with all the fullness of God. Now to Him who is able to do exceedingly abundantly above all that we ask or think, according to the power that works in us, to Him be glory in the church by Christ Jesus to all generation forever and ever. Amen) Ephesians 3:14-21

I pray you loved reading this book as much as I enjoyed writing it, together we can change the world one spine at a time, and heal the nations. (Jeff Trigo, D.C.)

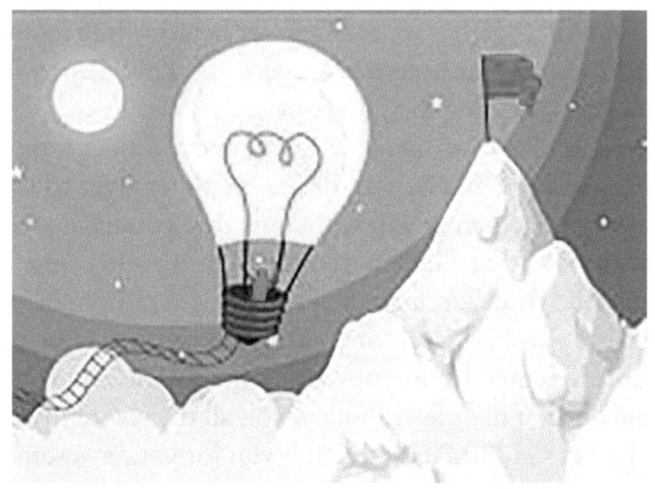

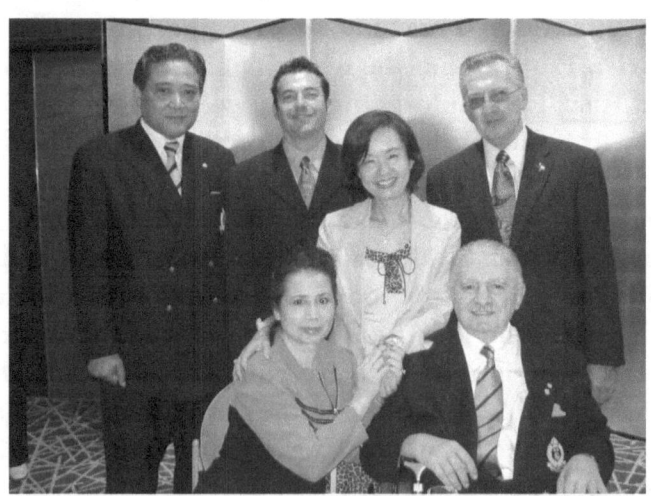

Dr. Iwama, Jeff Trigo, D.C., Dr. Richard Brassard, D.C.
Mrs. Iwama, Deloris Trigo, Robert F.S. Trigo, D.C.

About the Author

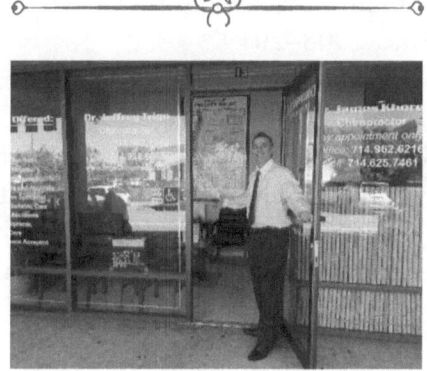

Jeffrey Trigo, DC, CME
Cleveland Chiropractic College LA Grad Aug 1999
20 year wellness practice serving Orange County and Los Angeles
for 20 years

Accomplishments:

- Doctorate of Chiropractic, Cleveland Chiropractic College, LA. August 1999
- Radiographic X-Ray Supervisor and Operator, California, 2000
- CME (Certified Medical Examiner) 2015
- Instructor with Japan Council on Chiropractic Education (JCCE) 2002
- Teacher of chiropractic technique with American Academy of Chiropractic Physicians (AACP) 2003-2012
- Director of Technique, Japan Chiropractic Association (JCA) since Sept 2007-2014

- Annual recipient from division of postgraduate studies, Texas Chiropractic College for Certificate of Appreciation for course instructor of technique JCA 9 years.

Experience:

- Doctor of Chiropractic and CEO of Trigo Health Chiropractic Inc., 2008–2019
- Doctor of Chiropractic at Huntington Beach Chiropractic 2007 to 2014
- Doctor of Chiropractic at Graham Chiropractic 1999-2007
- Cerrone Radiology, Huntington Beach 1991-1993 (Thermographic Technician)
- Trigo Thermographic Imaging and Analysis 1985-1988 (Thermographic Technician)

Awards/Activities

- Past president (three years) for Pierside Professionals LeTip of Huntington Beach
- Current President (sixteen years) www.SurfCityConnection.com Huntington Beach 2019
- Athlete and gold medal winner for Chiropractic Olympics, soccer, basketball 1996-99
- Awarded the Tri Extra-Miler Award for building class morale; active participation; enthusiasm for collage and chiropractic, and willingness to go the extra mile, 10-14-98
- Student Mentor Award, for outstanding contributions to the college and students, 1998
- Club Chiropractic award, for dedication to the continuance of chiropractic principle 1996
- Graduate 2010 "Parenting from the Heart" 18 hour comprehensive course
- Major supporter and organizer for Calvary Chapel Beachside Soup Kitchen (2008-2019)
- Head Coach AYSO Div. 56 U9 Boys Soccer, 2017

www.ingramcontent.com/pod-product-compliance
Lightning Source LLC
Chambersburg PA
CBHW061337280526
45784CB00001B/40